T0325382

ANNALS *of* THE NEW YORK ACADEMY OF SCIENCES

EDITOR-IN-CHIEF
Douglas Braaten

ASSOCIATE EDITOR
Rebecca E. Cooney

PROJECT MANAGER
Steven E. Bohall

EDITORIAL ADMINISTRATOR
Daniel J. Becker

Artwork and design by Ash Ayman Shairzay

The New York Academy of Sciences
7 World Trade Center
250 Greenwich Street, 40th Floor
New York, NY 10007-2157

annals@nyas.org
www.nyas.org/annals

The conference "Evolving Challenges in Promoting Cardiovascular Health" was jointly presented by the New York Academy of Sciences, "la Caixa" Foundation, and the International Center for Scientific Debate (ICSD) in Barcelona, Spain, 4-5 November 2011. The conference was generously supported by Academy Bronze Sponsors: Esteve, Ferrer, and Fundación Ramón Areces; and also by Academy Friend Sponsors: Bayer HealthCare, Laboratorios Servier España, Philips Healthcare, and Siemens, S.A. The conference was also supported by an independent education grant from Astellas Pharma Global Development and a strategic grant from the Edwards Lifesciences Fund. The conference was presented as part of the Academy's Translational Medicine Initiative, sponsored by the Josiah Macy Jr. Foundation and The Mushett Family Foundation. A selection of speaker presentations are available online at www.nyas.org/Cardiovascular-eB.

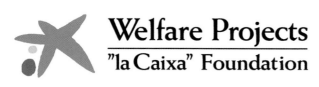

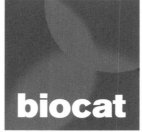

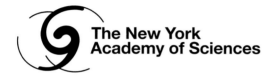

Published by Blackwell Publishing
On behalf of the New York Academy of Sciences

Boston, Massachusetts
2012

ANNALS *of* THE NEW YORK ACADEMY OF SCIENCES

VOLUME
1254

ISSUE

Evolving Challenges in Promoting Cardiovascular Health

ISSUE EDITOR
Valentin Fuster

Mount Sinai School of Medicine

TABLE OF CONTENTS

Ann. N.Y. Acad. Sci. ISSN 0077-8923

ANNALS OF THE NEW YORK ACADEMY OF SCIENCES
Issue: *Evolving Challenges in Promoting Cardiovascular Health*

Cardiovascular defense challenges at the basic, clinical, and population levels

Jason C. Kovacic,[1,2] Jose M. Castellano,[1,2] and Valentin Fuster[1,2,3]

[1]Zena and Michael A. Wiener Cardiovascular Institute, [2] Marie-Josée and Henry R. Kravis Cardiovascular Health Center, Mount Sinai School of Medicine, New York, New York. [3]Centro Nacional de Investigaciones Cardiovasculares (CNIC), Madrid, Spain

Address for correspondence: Valentin Fuster, M.D., Ph.D., Mount Sinai School of Medicine, One Gustave L. Levy Place, Box 1030, New York, NY 10029. valentin.fuster@mountsinai.org

Cardiovascular disease (CVD) is now the leading cause of mortality worldwide. Particularly in low and middle income countries, rapid urbanization and secondary factors, such as increasing obesity, poor diet, and lack of exercise, have combined to propel CVD into this position. Given the enormous scope of this problem and the complex cultural, societal, and political issues that are involved, an equally sophisticated and multipronged approach is required to combat CVD at the global level. In this review, we outline the basic, clinical, and population level challenges that we face in defending ourselves against this disease.

Keywords: cardiovascular defense; cardiovascular disease; socioeconomic status

It is well known that cardiovascular disease (CVD) is among the leading causes of mortality across the globe.[1,2] Somewhat encouragingly, the latest data from the United States indicate that from 1998 to 2008, the rate of death attributable to CVD declined 30.6%.[3] Nevertheless, U.S. mortality data for 2008 show that CVD continues to account for 1 of every 3 deaths.[3] Of this major cardiovascular burden of disease, atherosclerotic coronary artery disease (CAD) accounted for the major proportion of CVD morbidity, causing ~1 of every 6 deaths in the United States during this time.[3] Therefore, while inroads against CVD and CAD have been made, a great deal of work remains to be done. In this paper, we critically appraise the basic, clinical, and population-level challenges that remain to be addressed to adequately defend ourselves and the next generation against this epidemic.

Transition from complex CVD to promoting health

In decades past and to the present day, great effort has been devoted by both basic scientists and clinicians to pursuing the concept of the "vulnerable plaque." These vulnerable plaques are lipid-laden arterial atherosclerotic lesions that have an atten- uated overlying fibrous cap and that are prone to rupture and cause acute thrombotic arterial occlusion, which may lead to myocardial infarction or stroke.[4] Much attention was given to identifying these lesions in the hope that preventive interventions, such as the stenting of a nonobstructive but vulnerable plaque, would reduce subsequent clinical events. This has led to great advances in imaging techniques,[5–7] and the features of "high-risk vulnerable" (HRP) plaques that are prone to rupture and cause events have been well defined.[4] However, while there is no question that vulnerable plaques exist and that they can lead to fatal events, recent pivotal studies have helped us to understand that there is almost never a single vulnerable plaque in any given patient.[8] Moreover, while there may be multiple vulnerable plaques in any patient, the recent PROSPECT study taught us that predicting which of these will rupture and cause clinical events appears to be an exceptionally difficult task.[8] This has led to an important paradigm shift and change in our outlook toward CVD. Rather than thinking in terms of a "vulnerable plaque," we have gradually come to think in terms of the "vulnerable patient." That is to say, rupture-prone atherosclerotic plaques rarely exist in isolation, and rather than thinking

doi: 10.1111/j.1749-6632.2012.06495.x
Ann. N.Y. Acad. Sci. 1254 (2012) 1–6 © 2012 New York Academy of Sciences.

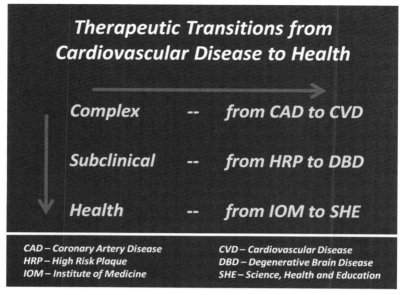

Figure 1. Overview of proposed therapeutic transitions from CAD to promoting global cardiovascular health. Adapted and reproduced with permission from Kovacic *et al.*[1]

about individual lesions, it is far more appropriate to consider the patient's entire vascular tree.

Concurrent to our appreciation of the "vulnerable patient" and as discussed elsewhere, it is also now increasingly recognized that degenerative brain disease (DBD) is intimately linked to the vasculature and overall burden of high risk plaque (HRP).[1,9] This HRP-DBD axis is operative across a very broad spectrum of disease, from macrovascular large vessel coronary or carotid occlusions leading MI or stroke, to microvascular small vessel changes causing dementia. Collectively, the critical importance of HRP with respect to brain, heart, kidney, and other organ function, together with the concept of the "vulnerable patient," is strong evidence that to make further progress in fighting this disease we must transition from considering primarily the coronary vessels (i.e., CAD), to looking at the entire patient in terms of systemic cardiovascular disease (CVD) (Fig. 1).

Basic challenges: aging and HDL-cholesterol pathways

With a few notable exceptions (see later), CVD is, in fact, a disease of aging. Advances in the last decade have yielded major breakthroughs in our understanding of the aging process at the genetic

and molecular level. As a focal point of these basic advances, the 2009 Nobel Prize was awarded for the discovery of telomeres and telomerase. Telomeres are sections of DNA at the ends of DNA strands that may become shortened with successive cellular division, while telomerase is an enzyme that aids in maintaining proper telomere length. As a key aspect of cellular aging, when telomeres reach a critically shortened length, cell division ceases and cellular senescence (from the Latin word *senex*, meaning old age or old man) then ensues. In simplistic terms, senescence is a form of "cellular hibernation" marked by growth arrest, resistance to apoptosis, and altered gene expression.[10,11] Furthermore, basic science insights from premature vascular aging disorders, such as Hutchinson-Gilford Progeria syndrome, have underscored the fact that cellular senescence is closely related to systemic aging.[11] Adequately defending ourselves against CVD will certainly be contingent upon a complete and proper understanding of the intricacies of telomere function.

Another pivotal basic advance has been our appreciation of the importance of reverse cholesterol transport.[12,13] In brief, this involves the transport and removal of cholesterol moieties from the periphery, and in particular from atherosclerotic plaques, back to the liver. Once at the liver, the cholesterol moieties may be excreted and eliminated. This process is largely under the purview of high-density lipoprotein (HDL) cholesterol,[14] and has seen intense efforts directed toward therapeutically raising the levels of this lipoprotein. Although other agents exist, the cholesteryl ester transfer protein (CETP) inhibitors are the prototypical drugs developed to promote reverse cholesterol transport. CETP, a plasma protein, facilitates the shuttling of lipids and triglycerides between transporting lipoprotein particles. Clinical trials with anacetrapib, a CETP inhibitor, successfully lowered the levels of low-density lipoprotein (LDL) cholesterol while raising HDL cholesterol by 138%.[15] Our group has recently reported a major study of another CETP inhibitor, dalcetrapib. In this 130 patient, double-blind, multicenter trial, the use of dalcetrapib was associated with likely beneficial vascular effects, including a reduction in vessel enlargement over 24 months. Although not powered for clinical endpoints, there was no difference in event rates between the placebo and dalcetrapib groups.[16] The much larger dal-OUTCOMES study, with >15,000 patients, is now investigating the efficacy of this agent for reducing CVD events in patients that recently suffered from an index acute coronary syndrome.[17]

Certainly, a vast number of basic science discoveries have been made that have advanced our knowledge of CVD. However, the examples of telomeres/senescence and reverse cholesterol transport illustrate the point that the successful and timely clinical translation of basic discoveries is vital to defending ourselves against CVD.

Clinical challenges: the HRP initiative subclinical study and the polypill

Although we may be in the process of transitioning from considering CAD to systemic CVD, and from the vulnerable plaque to the vulnerable patient, a lingering question that remains to be properly addressed is: who is at risk for CVD? At present, risk assessment is typically performed by simple algorithms, such as the Framingham Risk Score, with simple online tools readily available to calculate 10-year risk of CAD-related adverse events (http://www.mdcalc.com/framingham-cardiac-risk-score). Although these tools can give a reasonable estimate of 5- or 10-year risk for

events, they have very limited utility for identifying asymptomatic patients who are at risk for near-term CVD-related events.[18] Aggressive primary prevention is likely to avert major morbidity and mortality in patients at risk for near-term events, and a window of opportunity exists for therapeutic intervention. In an attempt to define novel and efficacious approaches to identify and treat those at risk for near-term events, the High Risk Plaque (HRP) Bioimage study was recently initiated.[18] Over 7,500 patients at-risk for CVD events, but without manifestations of atherothrombotic disease, were entered into this study. Subjects underwent comprehensive baseline assessment, which included determination of CVD risk factors, quantification of coronary artery calcification by computed tomography, measurement of intima-media thickness, carotid and abdominal aortic artery ultrasound, and ankle-brachial index assessment. Participants with one or more abnormal results in these screening tests underwent additional imaging evaluation. The trial is now in an active follow-up phase, and initial results will soon be at hand. Importantly, this study will identify all CVD-related events, including DBD and stroke, and will permit global measures of CVD, burden of HRP and even the genetics of this disease to be correlated and explored in depth. By arming ourselves with this information, clinicians will be far better informed to make proactive treatment decisions.

At its core, the HRP study is driving at optimizing primary prevention. Although identifying at-risk patients is one aspect of this problem, many other challenges remain to be addressed at the patient and clinical level before we can prevent CVD. As the complexity of medical treatments continue to increase, the adherence of patients to these sometimes daunting poly-pharmaceutical therapeutic regimens is a growing concern. Indeed, nonadherence to prescribed therapies may occur in ~50% of patients,[19,20] accounting for $290 billion of U.S. annual health care expenditure.[21] Aligned with transitioning toward treating systemic CVD, the drive toward the widespread implementation of a polypill as a primary preventive agent or secondary treatment is gaining in momentum. The polypill has multiple potential advantages for the patient, including increased convenience and adherence, but also decreased cost. The polypill can combine several agents that tackle platelet adhesiveness (aspirin), blood pressure (ACE inhibitor, thiazide diuretic), lipid levels (statin), and other aspects of CVD primary risk management or secondary treatment. Recent estimates suggest that widespread polypill use by U.S. adults aged ≥55 years may prevent 3.2 million CAD events and 1.7 million strokes over 10 years.[22] Several randomized clinical trials of the polypill are now underway aiming to define their potential effects on CVD risk factors and clinical outcomes.[22] Nevertheless, as the polypill potentially moves into clinical practice, physicians will need to remain cognizant of the need to balance the merits of the inexpensive but relatively fixed combinations available via polypills, with the need to individualize therapies to the particular needs of each patient.

These are but a few examples of the many challenges we face and progress being made at the clinical level in defending ourselves against CVD. Other notable (but by no means all) clinical challenges include achieving the implementation of guideline recommendations, moving from paper-based to electronic medical record systems, improving communication, and adopting a team-based approach to health care delivery.

Population challenges: IOM report, UN and chronic diseases, and the SHE initiative

Defending ourselves against CVD is a global concern. Although in Western societies, mortality rates from CVD may have improved marginally, in low- and middle-income countries (LMICs), the situation remains grim. In certain LMICs up to 75% of deaths are attributable to CVD.[23] This is due to a complex set of interacting factors that include rapid modernization and "Westernization," inadequate availability of nutritious foods and poor diet, lack of exercise, high prevalence of tobacco use, and lack of attention to other CVD risk factors (hypertension, diabetes, hyperlipidemia). The Institute of Medicine (IOM; the health arm of the U.S. National Academy of Sciences) recently began to engage these issues by establishing a high-level committee to review the relevant factors affecting global CVD health. This led to the tabling of a raft of initiatives focusing on tackling CVD in LMICs, titled "Promoting Cardiovascular Health in the Developing World: A Critical Challenge to Achieve Global Health."[1,24,25] As shown in Figure 2, the report provides a compre-

hensive framework for attacking the global threat of CVD.

This has been echoed by the General Assembly of the United Nations (UN). In an historic two-day meeting in September 2011, noncommunicable diseases were deemed a development challenge of "epidemic proportions." The World Health Organization chief stated that the "meeting must be [a]wake-up call—a watershed event that replaces ignorance and inertia with awareness and right actions."[26] Member states signed a declaration that addresses tobacco, industrially produced trans-fats in foods, and several other key issues related to the world's leading noncommunicable diseases, and CVD in particular. Further consensus was reached as to the root causes driving the increase of noncommunicable diseases: the use of tobacco, excess alcohol consumption, poor-quality food, lack of exercise, and lack of access to healthcare services and medicines.[26] Although this UN meeting and the IOM document have outlined the problems and the road forward, the hard task must now begin of actually implementing these recommendations and changes.

As an extension of some of these challenges we face in enacting population level changes, a major hurdle to be addressed is the willingness of patients to adopt healthy behavioral patterns. Finding ways to motivate people to stop smoking and to "move (exercise) more and eat less" is critical. It is our personal belief and experience that teaching healthy habits from a young age is the key to success. The notion of health education and motivation among young persons is encapsulated by the SHE initiative: The Foundation for Science, Health, and Education. SHE is a multifaceted program that is aiming to better educate children and young adults about how to live a healthier lifestyle. Projects run by SHE include a preschool trial to promote cardiovascular health in 6,000 children in Columbia (enrollment complete) and now a planned extension of that study to 25,000 participants, various educational children's books, a "Healthy Habits Campaign" involving youth sports programs in Spain, studies of changing cardiovascular risks in Grenada with rapid modernization, and multinational studies involving the polypill based in Europe and New York.[27] This type of work being undertaken by the SHE foundation, in conjunction with a great deal of other work that remains to be done, should see the next

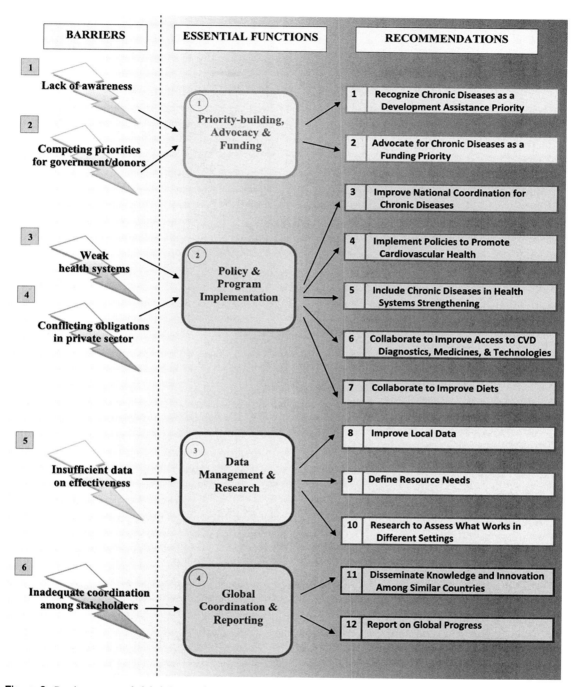

Figure 2. Barriers to control global CVD and essential functions and recommendations to overcome those barriers arising from the Institute of Medicine document "Promoting Cardiovascular Health in the Developing World: A Critical Challenge to Achieve Global Health." Figure reproduced with permission from Fuster *et al.*[24]

generation far better equipped to make healthy life choices.

Conclusions

Cardiovascular health is a major global concern that cannot be effectively tackled by any single therapy, intervention, or initiative. From the study of vulnerable atherosclerotic plaques to support from the United Nations, major transitions are in progress that will aid in managing this problem (Fig. 1). Looking ahead, a concerted effort across multiple disciplines, and a determination to move forward and overcome inevitable obstacles will be required if we are to effectively defend ourselves and the next generation against this disease.

Acknowledgments

No specific funding or grant was used to prepare this manuscript. Jason Kovacic is supported by National Institutes of Health Grant 1K08HL111330–01.

Conflicts of interest

The authors declare no conflicts of interest.

References

1. Kovacic, J.C. *et al.* 2011. From treating complex coronary artery disease to promoting cardiovascular health: therapeutic transitions and challenges, 2010–2020. *Clin. Pharmacol. Ther.* **90:** 509–518.
2. Kovacic, J.C. *et al.* 2011. Cellular senescence, vascular disease, and aging: part 1 of a 2-part review. *Circulation* **123:** 1650–1660.
3. Roger, V.L. *et al.* 2012. Heart disease and stroke statistics–2012 update: a report from the American Heart Association. *Circulation* **125:** e2–e220.
4. Moreno, P.R. *et al.* 2009. Promoting mechanisms of vascular health: circulating progenitor cells, angiogenesis, and reverse cholesterol transport. *J. Am. Coll. Cardiol.* **53:** 2315–2323.
5. Rudd, J.H. *et al.* 2010. Imaging atherosclerotic plaque inflammation by fluorodeoxyglucose with positron emission tomography: ready for prime time? *J. Am. Coll. Cardiol.* **55:** 2527–2535.
6. Underhill, H.R. *et al.* 2010. MRI of carotid atherosclerosis: clinical implications and future directions. *Nat. Rev. Cardiol.* **7:** 165–173.
7. Klink, A. *et al.* 2011. Diagnostic and therapeutic strategies for small abdominal aortic aneurysms. *Nat. Rev. Cardiol.* **8:** 338–347.
8. Stone, G.W. *et al.* 2011. A prospective natural-history study of coronary atherosclerosis. *N. Engl. J. Med.* **364:** 226–235.
9. Kovacic, J.C. *et al.* 2011. Cellular senescence, vascular disease, and aging: part 2 of a 2-part review: clinical vascular disease in the elderly. *Circulation.* **123:** 1900–1910.
10. Campisi, J. *et al.* 2007. Cellular senescence: when bad things happen to good cells. *Nat. Rev. Mol. Cell. Biol.* **8:** 729–740.
11. Olive, M. *et al.* 2010. Cardiovascular pathology in Hutchinson-Gilford progeria: correlation with the vascular pathology of aging. *Arterioscler. Thromb. Vasc. Biol.* **30:** 2301–2309.
12. Fayad, Z.A. *et al.* 2011. Safety and efficacy of dalcetrapib on atherosclerotic disease using novel non-invasive multimodality imaging (dal-PLAQUE): a randomised clinical trial. *Lancet.* **378:** 1547–1559.
13. Fayad, Z.A. *et al.* 2011. Rationale and design of dal-PLAQUE: a study assessing efficacy and safety of dalcetrapib on progression or regression of atherosclerosis using magnetic resonance imaging and 18F-fluorodeoxyglucose positron emission tomography/computed tomography. *Am. Heart J.* **162:** 214–221 e2.
14. Navab, M. *et al.* 2011. HDL and cardiovascular disease: atherogenic and atheroprotective mechanisms. *Nat. Rev. Cardiol.* **8:** 222–232.
15. Cannon, C.P. *et al.* 2010. Safety of anacetrapib in patients with or at high risk for coronary heart disease. *N. Engl. J. Med.* **363:** 2406–2415.
16. Fayad, Z.A. *et al.* 2011. Safety and efficacy of dalcetrapib on atherosclerotic disease using novel non-invasive multimodality imaging (dal-PLAQUE): a randomised clinical trial. *Lancet.* **378:** 1547–1559.
17. Soe, K. *et al.* 2011. Cardiovascular risk reduction via increasing HDL cholesterol: the promise of the dal-OUTCOMES Trial. *Curr. Diab. Rep.* **11:** 4–6.
18. Muntendam, P. *et al.* 2010. The BioImage Study: novel approaches to risk assessment in the primary prevention of atherosclerotic cardiovascular disease–study design and objectives. *Am. Heart J.* **160:** 49–57 e1.
19. Boden, W.E. *et al.* 2007. Optimal medical therapy with or without PCI for stable coronary disease. *N. Engl. J. Med.* **356:** 1503–1516.
20. Frye, R.L. *et al.* 2009. A randomized trial of therapies for type 2 diabetes and coronary artery disease. *N. Engl. J. Med.* **360:** 2503–2515.
21. Epstein, R.S. 2011. Medication adherence: hope for improvement? *Mayo Clin. Proc.* **86:** 268–270.
22. Muntner, P. *et al.* 2011. Projected impact of polypill use among US adults: medication use, cardiovascular risk reduction, and side effects. *Am. Heart J.* **161:** 719–725.
23. World Health Organization. 2009. World Health Statistics. Available at: http://www.who.int/research/en. Accessed 10 May 2011.
24. Fuster, V. *et al.* 2011. Promoting global cardiovascular health: moving forward. *Circulation* **123:** 1671–1678.
25. Kishore, S.P. *et al.* 2011. Promoting global cardiovascular health ensuring access to essential cardiovascular medicines in low- and middle-income countries. *J. Am. Coll. Cardiol.* **57:** 1980–1987.
26. Non-communicable diseases deemed development challenge of 'Epidemic Proportions'. Available at http://www.un.org/News/Press/docs/2011/ga11138.doc.htm. Accessed 16 Jan 2011.
27. Taylor, J. 2011. Science is the fundamental building block for every project in The Foundation for Science, Health, and Education (SHE). *Eur. Heart J.* **32:** 662–663.

Ann. N.Y. Acad. Sci. ISSN 0077-8923

Plaque neovascularization: defense mechanisms, betrayal, or a war in progress

Pedro R. Moreno, Meeranani Purushothaman, and K-Raman Purushothaman

Zena and Michael A. Wiener Cardiovascular Institute, and the Marie-Josee and Henry R. Kravis Cardiovascular Health Center, Mount Sinai School of Medicine, New York, New York

Address for correspondence: Pedro R. Moreno, M.D., Professor of Medicine/Cardiology, Mount Sinai School of Medicine, Box 1030, New York, NY 10029. pedro.moreno@mountsinai.org

Angiogenesis is induced from sprouting of preexisting endothelial cells leading to neovascularization. Imbalance in the angiogenic and antiangiogenic mediators triggers angiogenesis, which may be physiological in the normal state or pathological in malignancy and atherosclerosis. Physiologic angiogenesis is instrumental for restoration of vessel wall normoxia and resolution inflammation, leading to atherosclerosis regression. However, pathological angiogenesis enhances disease progression, increasing macrophage infiltration and vessel wall thickness, perpetuating hypoxia and necrosis. In addition, thin-walled fragile neovessels may rupture, leading to intraplaque hemorrhage. Lipid-rich red blood cell membranes and free hemoglobin are detrimental to plaque composition, increasing inflammation, lipid core expansion, and oxidative stress. In addition, associated risk factors that include polymorphysms in the haptoglobin genotype and diabetes mellitus may modulate the features of plaque vulnerability. This review will focus on physiological and pathological angiogenesis in atherosclerosis and summarizes the current status of anti-vascular endothelial growth factor (VEGF) therapy, microvascular rarefaction, and possible statin-mediated effects in atherosclerosis neovascularization.

Keywords: angiogenesis; hypoxia; atherosclerosis; neovascularization

Introduction

Evolving complications of cardiovascular disease (CVD) contribute to be leading causes of morbidity and mortality in the world. However, the tremendous investment in prevention and therapy is now providing encouraging results. Within the last decade, the number of acute myocardial infarctions has declined by 23%, and the percentage of sudden cardiac deaths attributable to CVD declined by 31%.[1,2] This decrease in CVD may be partially explained by disease regression, and plaque neovascularization may be at the center of this process.

In the absence of disease, the normal vessel wall receives oxygen (O_2) by diffusion from the lumen. As extracellular matrix accumulates in the intima, O_2 diffusion becomes insufficient to nurture the vessel wall, mostly at the intimomedial junction. From the fatty streak to the advanced fibroatheroma, the atherosclerotic lesion is governed by metabolically active cells that require O_2 to live. With progressively reduced concentrations of O_2, aerobic cells express hypoxic-inducible factor (HIF) to create new vessels and counteract the unfavorable balance between O_2 offer and demand.[3] This biological defense mechanism to prevent hypoxia-induced necrosis and to maintain tissue integrity is known as *physiological angiogenesis*.

Plaque neovascularization as a defense mechanism: physiological angiogenesis

Angiogenesis is fundamental for development, reproduction, and repair. Angiogenesis is responsible for the resolution of wound healing, endometrial growth during the menstrual cycle, tissue grafting, inflammation, and hypoxia. These and other stimuli trigger the "angiogenic switch," a state in which angiogenic factors predominate over angiostatic factors. Endothelial cells (ECs) are responsible for angiogenesis. Regulated by multiple molecular

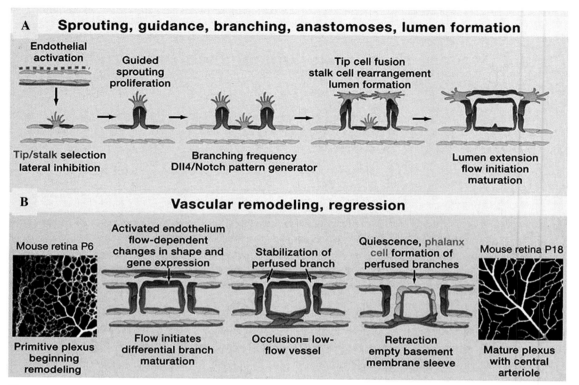

Figure 1. Hallmarks of neovessel formation. (A) Steps of vessel sprouting: (1) tip/stalk cell selection; (2) tip cell navigation and stalk cell proliferation; (3) branching coordination; (4) stalk elongation, tip cell fusion, and lumen formation; and (5) perfusion and vessel maturation. (B) Sequential steps of vascular remodeling from a primitive (left box) toward a stabilized and mature vascular plexus (right box) include adoption of a quiescent endothelial phalanx phenotype, basement membrane deposition, pericyte coverage, and branch regression. Reproduced with permission from Potente *et al.*[5]

mechanisms, this angiogenic switch includes the initiation, activation, and migration of ECs followed by tube formation and finally microvessel stabilization (Fig. 1). The main mechanism of angiogenesis is vessel sprouting. Although other mechanisms, such as vessel splitting, intussusception, or stimulation of vessel expansion by circulating precursor cells,[4,5] may also contribute, EC sprouting is by far the predominant pathway for angiogenesis.[5] ECs are liberated from the basement membrane by detachment from mural cells. This initial process is mediated by matrix metalloproteinases such as MMP1. These proteolytic enzymes liberate proangiogenic growth factors.[5,6] ECs then become motile and invasive by tip and stalk cell formation. Filopodia guide these tip cells for tube formation, with final stabilization of the endothelial layer (Fig. 1). Oxygen perfusion is then restored to hypoxic areas followed by tissue repair.

Physiological angiogenesis is usually focal, self-limited in time, with days (ovulation), weeks (wound healing), or months (placentation).[7] A fundamental concept of physiological angiogenesis relies on its total reversibility after resolution of the condition that triggered angiogenesis. In atherosclerosis, hypoxia (and other triggers) may be responsible for angiogenesis. After resolution of hypoxia and restitution of homeostasis, neovessels are not needed anymore, closing the circle with angiogenesis involution. This physiological response to injury leads to proper healing of the vessel wall, as seen in disease regression.

Hypoxia and angiogenesis
Atherosclerotic plaque progression is characterized by inflammation (increased O_2 demand) and intimal thickness (decreased O_2 supply), resulting in hypoxia, the most potent trigger of angiogenesis.[8]

Studies in atherosclerotic rabbits clearly show increased necrosis, fat deposition, and macrophage infiltration co-localizing with areas of hypoxia.[9] Metabolic analysis displays severe ATP depletion in macrophages, glucose depletion, and increased lactate (anaerobic) metabolism. In humans, the hypoxia marker pimonidazole co-localized with areas of macrophage infiltration, angiogenesis, and thrombus in carotid plaques before surgical repair.[10] Using oxygen microelectrodes in atherosclerotic vessels, mid-regions of the aortic arch and femoral arteries showed a significant gradient when compared to adventitia. These plaques displayed levels of oxygen as low as 0–15 mmHg, compared to 50 mmHg close to the adventitia or arterial lumen.[3] In addition, inflamed areas are virtually always hypoxic because of its high metabolic demand. Lipid deposition will trigger activated macrophage infiltration, creating a cycle of inflammation, hypoxia, and angiogenesis. As such, plaque neovascularization is a defense mechanism that usually co-localizes with macrophages and may be used as a surrogate marker for inflammation.

Although plaque thickness plays a role, inflammatory cell content is the most important determinant of hypoxia. When oxygen tension decreases from normal levels (20–100 mmHg) to less than 10 mmHg, hypoxia triggers a molecular pathway mostly mediated by HIF-1 alpha (HIF-1α). The HIF transcription factor is composed of two subunits, a ubiquitous HIF-1β subunit and a hypoxic responsive subunit HIF-1α.[11] Migration of the HIF-1α-β dimer to the nucleus initiates transcriptional upregulation of multiple angiogenic factors, including vascular endothelial growth factor (VEGF). Under normoxic conditions, the oxygen-sensing enzymes prolyl hydroxylase domain (PHD) proteins 1–3 hydroxylate HIF-1α, and HIF-2α.[12] Once hydroxylated, HIFs are targeted for proteasomal degradation.[13] Hypoxia suppresses PHD activity and stabilizes HIFs. Hypoxia and inflammation are closely intertwined, and several hypoxia-activated genes are regulated by proinflammatory cytokines that results in the vasa vasorum proliferation and invasion.[14,15] In the atherosclerotic plaque, hypoxia- and inflammation-mediated increase of HIF-1α expression may act through two different mechanisms. In macrophages, an increase in HIF-1α activity may induce angiogenic and inflammatory factors that lead to immature neovessel formation, resulting in

intraplaque hemorrhage (IPH) and plaque destabilization. In ECs, PHD-mediated hydroxylation of HIF-1α may inhibit angiogenesis, reducing IPH and leading to plaque stabilization. Of significant relevance, heterozygous deficiency of PHD2 restores tumor oxygenation and inhibits metastasis via endothelial normalization.[16] Although hypoxia is by far the most studied trigger of angiogenesis, recent data show that oxidized low-density lipoprotein (oxLDL) can increase the expression of HIF-1 and VEGF in normoxic conditions. In addition, oxLDL can also induce endothelial proliferation in an *in vivo* model of matrigel tube formation.[17]

Physiological angiogenesis and resolution of atheroma

As a defense mechanism, physiological angiogenesis may be a functional pathway for macrophages to remove cholesterol from the plaque.[18] Studies evaluating blood flow across the vessel wall documented 10-fold increase in transaortic wall microspheres within vasa vasorum in primates with atherosclerosis.[19] Our group documented histological evidence of macrophages and T cell trafficking within microvessels in human atherosclerotic plaques[20] (Fig. 2). Studies quantifying plaque composition by planimetry show significant reduction of lipid content in fibrocalcific plaques.[21] Simultaneously, fibrocalcific plaques are characterized by the lowest microvessel content, suggesting involution of angiogenesis after resolution of the atheromatous component in advanced human plaques.[22] With the above observations, our group postulated that functional angiogenesis contributes to the removal of intimal fat when the concentration of LDL is lower in the neovessel circulation than in the intima (LDL concentration gradient).[23] This observation is supported by multiple studies showing reduced plaque burden with aggressive statin therapy.[24–26] More recently, the SATURN study documented plaque regression in up to 68% of patients treated with aggressive statin therapy.[27] As a result, the resolution of hypercholesterolemia is associated with plaque regression in humans.

Experimental atherosclerosis follows the same pattern. Atherosclerotic lesions of apolipoprotein E knockout (Apo E$^{-/-}$) mice exposed to low levels of cholesterol experience plaque regression. The mechanisms involved in plaque regression were studied using aortic plaques from the Apo E$^{-/-}$

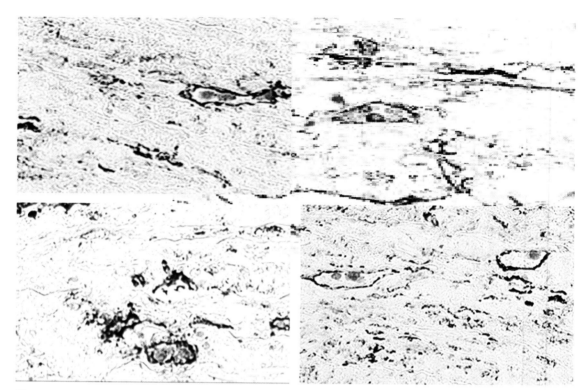

Figure 2. Neovessels with intraluminal macrophages. Double-label immunochemistry images (40× magnification) in four panels. Shows bicolor contrasting microvessels in cross-sections identified with the monoclonal EC marker CD34 linked to a blue chromogen, and inflammatory cells identified with a combined macrophage/T cell marker CD68–CD3 linked to a red chromogen. This image depicts the alternate pathway of inflammatory cell trafficking through the microvessel.

mice transplanted into wild-type mice.[28] M2 macrophages and dendritic cells migrate through adventitial lymph vessels to local lymph nodes in a process that is dependent on the chemotactic ligands of the G protein–coupled chemokine receptor 7 (CCR7).[29] A series of insightful observations in this transplant model promoted CCR7 as the pivotal molecule of plaque regression.[30,31] The molecular mechanisms involved the liver X receptor (responsible for the HDL-dependent reverse cholesterol transport), the MERTK engulfment receptor, and others.[32,33] Using this transplant model, aggressive statin therapy promoted CD68+ cell emigration increasing transcriptional activity and chromatin organization at the CCR7 promoter.[28]

These observations have been recently challenged by another model of plaque regression. The Apo E–encoding adenoviral vector model identified a different pattern of macrophage removal in the same Apo E−/− mice model. Restitution of the Apo E protein normalizes plasma cholesterol to wild-type levels and increases HDL levels fourfold.[34] Within four weeks of therapy, a 72% reduction in macrophage content was observed *independent* from CCR7.[34] Most importantly, a marked inhibition of macrophage recruitment from circulating monocytes was achieved by significant reductions in endothelial adhesion molecules. As a result, suppressed monocyte recruitment, rather than CCR7 efferocytosis, may be the predominant mechanism in plaque regression. In addition, local proliferation of M2 macrophages may contribute to plaque regression be responsible for clearance of apoptotic cells and TGF-β–mediated collagen synthesis.[35]

Plaque neovascularization as a morbid condition: pathological angiogenesis

Pathological angiogenesis evolves as an acute and sustained angiogenic response arising from the uncontrolled EC stimulation.[36] This may be induced by perturbation of the normal physiological mechanisms, in both the initiation and the

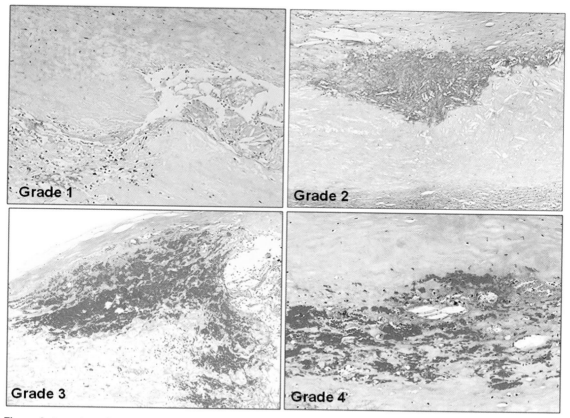

Figure 3. Intraplaque hemorrhage grading. Hematoxylin and eosin stain sections (20× magnification) identifying IPH, defined as red blood cell extravasation with fibrin deposition within the necrotic core. IPH was graded from 1 to 4 according to the IPH area occupied within the lipid core (1 = 25%; 2 = 50%; 3 = 75%; and 4 = 100% of lipid core).

resolution phases.[37] The initiation phase of physiological angiogenesis is characterized by sprouting, tube formation, and pericyte-mediated stabilization. Resolution of hypoxia downregulates VEGF expression, increasing endothelial angiopoietin 1, PDGF, and TGF-β1, leading to the resolution phase, which involves a cascade of molecular signaling.[5] In contrast, during pathological angiogenesis there is a failure of resolution phase due to sustained immune cell-mediating cytokines, which triggers the ECs to persistent synthesis of VEGF, leading to persistence of angiogenic stimuli.[36,38]

IPH

IPH is defined as the extravasation of red blood cells (RBCs) admixed with fibrin and platelet matrix within the plaque. The intensity of IPH varies from mild to severe, and our group has classified IPH from grade 1 to grade 4 based on percentage area of hemorrhage occupied in the plaque[39] (Fig. 3). IPH also contributes to increase in plaque burden. This may explain the rapid progression of advanced, high-risk plaques, in which up to 40% display IPH.[40] Three fundamental aspects are responsible for extravasation of RBCs: the microendothelium is poorly formed with EC gap junctions; basement membrane of neovessels are devoid of strong structural integrity; and most of the neovessels lack mural cell covering by pericytes or smooth muscle cells.[41] Furthermore, neovessels lack the background support within the matrix. Increased expression of VEGF liberated by macrophages will increase permeability of neovessels.[42] RBC membranes contain 40% more cholesterol than any other cell in the body. As a result, IPH is a major source for lipid core expansion, as previously reported.[41,43] Plaques with IPH are associated with rapid progression of disease, repeat hemorrhage, and clinical events.[44] Carotid plaques with 50–79% stenosis are usually treated medically because of the low incidence of clinical events. However, IPH dramatically changes the natural history of these nonobstructive plaques, with a fivefold increased incidence of stroke.[45] RBC extravasation and membrane lysis releases free hemoglobin (Hb). Extra corpuscular Hb triggers a Fenton reaction, generating reactive oxygen species (ROS), scavenging nitric oxide, and generating ferric iron by oxidation.[46–49]

Defense mechanism against IPH: the haptoglobin protein

Haptoglobin (Hp) binds Hb,[50,51] preventing the deleterious effects of free heme.[52] Mammals, which are protected from atherosclerosis, are classically homozygous for Hp with only one allele at the chromosomal locus. Humans, the only mammal that suffers from atherosclerosis, developed two alleles (1 and 2) at the Hp locus at chromosome 16q22.[53] The Hp 2 allele is structurally and functionally different from the Hp 1 allele; as a result, Hp 1 (monovalent) and Hp 2 (bivalent) allelic proteins are also different.[54] The Hp 2–2 genotype is an inferior protein with increased ROS generation, stimulating a proinflammatory and prooxidative phenotype.[54–56] Multiple studies have shown that patients with Hp 2–2 genotype have increased risk for cardiovascular events, both in primary and in secondary prevention.[51,57,58]

Clearance of free Hb from the atherosclerotic plaque: CD163 and HO-1 protein

Clearance of the Hb–Hp complex is mediated by the macrophage scavenger receptor CD163.[59–61] Also known as the Hb receptor, CD163 mediates the endocytosis of Hb–Hp complex, counteracting Hb-induced oxidative tissue damage.[62] CD163 is expressed by resident tissue macrophages and on infiltrating monocytes during the resolution phase of inflammatory reactions. CD163 expression is enhanced by anti-inflammatory mediators, such as interleukin-10, supporting the notion that CD163 is linked to an anti-inflammatory macrophage function.[62,63] Furthermore, binding of Hb–Hp complex to CD163 also elicits induction of heme oxygenase-1 (HO-1), a major cytoprotective enzyme. HO-1 degrades heme to carbon monoxide (CO), biliverdin, and ferrous iron.[64–66] All three molecules are known to be anti-inflammatory and antiatherosclerotic. This may be of special relevance for patients with

diabetes mellitus (DM). Human plaques from DM with Hp 2–2 genotype showed decreased CD163 protein and mRNA expression when compared to Hp 1–1 genotype.[54] The signaling protein, protein kinase C (PKC) is increased, upregulating the expression of proteases in the presence of increased oxidative stress.[67] PKC cleaves the scavenger receptor CD163 and leads to increased shedding of CD163. In addition, the expression of HO-1 mRNA may also be reduced in DM patients with Hp 2–2 genotype.[68]

Neovascularization in DM

Plaque inflammation, neovascularization, and IPH are increased in patients with DM.[69,70] DM is associated with a prooxidative and inflammatory state leading to systemic elevation of TNF-α, VEGF, PDGF, IGF-1, IL-1, AGE, and RAGE levels.[71–73] Most importantly, the endothelial adhesion molecules and cytokines are up-regulated leading to increased leucocytes emigration and monocyte/macrophage influx and subintimal proliferation favoring a neovessel proliferative mileu. Increased IPH with decreased Hb clearance will lead to iron deposition in DM. Experimental Hp2–2 transgenic mouse showed significant increase in iron deposition in the setting of DM.[74] Recently, our group documented increased iron deposition in human DM plaques with Hp 2–2 genotype.[75]

Therapeutic implications

Antiangiogenic therapy proved to be successful to reduce atheroma volume and macropahge infiltration in experimental atherosclerosis.[76] Furthermore, approaches aimed at blocking vessel growth provide excellent results in age-related macular degeneration (AMD) and cancer therapy.[77] Bevacizumab, a humanized variant of a VEGF-specific neutralizing monoclonal antibody,[78,79] was approved by the Food and Drug Administration (FDA) for cancer therapy. Other FDA-approved antiangiogenic agents for cancer treatment include sorafenib and sunitinib.[80–85]

A recent strategy for atherosclerotic treatment showed $\alpha_v\beta_3$ integrin-targeted paramagnetic nanoparticles containing the antiangiogenic drug fumagillin allowed site-specific delivery of drug to plaque-associated neovascularization at a fraction of the levels used for systemic treatments and

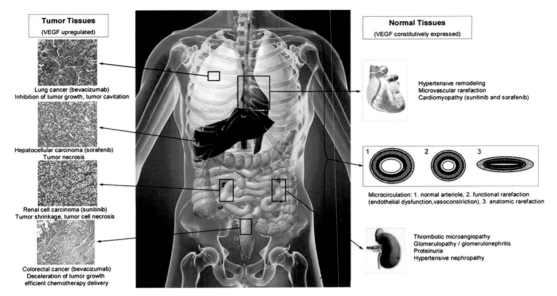

Figure 4. Differential effects of anti-VEGF therapy on tumor cells and normal cells. VEGF inhibition by the approved anti-VEGF therapies has differential effects on the VEGF–VEGFR axis in tumor cells and normal tissues. In noncancer tissues, endothelial dysfunction and microvascular rarefaction set the stage for the development of hypertension, cardiomyopathy, and thrombotic microangiopathy and proteinuria in the kidney (histologic pictures courtesy of Dr. Elsa Sotelo, University of Texas at Houston). Reproduced with permission from Vaklavas *et al.*[87]

provided integrated noninvasive monitoring of plaque microvascular density as a surrogate marker of atherosclerosis.[86]

Anti-VEGF therapy

Bevacizumab has been extensively used in several clinical trials. In addition to standard chemotherapy, bevacizumab has improved survival in patients with metastatic colorectal, lung, or breast cancer.[87] Recent phase III clinical trials have shown that treatment with pegaptanib, an anti-VEGF aptamer, and ranibizumab, an anti-VEGF antibody fragment, can maintain or improve vision in AMD patients,[88–90] indicating antiangiogenic therapy also "normalizes" and stabilizes immature vasculature in the eye. It is possible that anti-VEGF therapy may decrease the recruitment of leukocytes to the atherosclerotic plaque, decreasing the inflammatory response. Selective blockade of VEGF receptor 1 (VEGFR-1) by either anti-VEGFR-1 antibodies or antiplacenta-growth factor antibodies could also promote vessel normalization while avoiding systemic toxicities.[81] However, the potential benefits of antiangiogenic therapy in atherosclerosis may be limited by side effects and increased cardiovascular events.[91–93]

Cardiovascular risk and anti-VEGF therapy

The main cardiovascular-adverse effects of these compounds include proteinuria, hypertension, left ventricular systolic dysfunction, and thrombotic complications. In addition, data from five randomized clinical trials in patients with metastatic carcinomas demonstrated more arterial thromboembolic events in patients treated with conventional therapy plus bevacizumab (anti-VEGF) group than in the conventional therapy-only group (i.e., non-antiangiogenic). As atherosclerosis itself is an important risk factor for arterial thromboembolic events, these data underscore the dangers of using systemic high-dose antiangiogenic agents in patients with underlying atherosclerotic disease.[94] The mechanisms responsible for this are unclear but may involve selective deleterious effect on healthy endothelium, including microvascular rarefaction.

Anti-VEGF therapy and microvascular tarefaction

VEGF signaling in normal cardiac physiology extends beyond angiogenesis and mediates important compensatory responses to stress and injury.[87] Inhibition of VEGF signaling with anti-VEGF therapies leads to endothelial dysfunction, promoting extinction of the small blood vessels and compromising physiologic regulation of microcirculation. This important pathological side effect of anti-VEGF therapy is known as microvascular rarefaction (Fig. 4). This sets the stage for development of hypertension, cardiomyopathy, and thrombotic microangiopathy.

Anticholesterol therapy

Hydroxy-3-methylglutaryl coenzyme A (HMG-CoA) reductase inhibitors have been successfully used in human atherosclerosis with impressive reductions in cardiovascular events.[95,96] Evidence is mounting on the pleiotropic effects of statins, which include quenching of NF-κB and increasing PPARγ as well as PPARγ activation. These processes affect not only vascular inflammation but also angiogenesis. The effects of statins in atherosclerosis neovascularization are evolving.[97] A recent report indicates that atorvastatin treatment inhibits plaque development by reducing adventitial neovasculaization in Apo E–deficient mice independent of cholesterol levels.[26]

Antagonists of the angiotensin pathway reduce cardiovascular mortality and have recognized moderate antiangiogenic actions, but it is not clear whether the two effects are related,[97,98] and further studies are needed.

Conclusions

Atherosclerosis is characterized by inflammation and intimal thickness, increasing oxygen demand, and reducing supply. Hypoxia triggers a series of transcriptional processes mostly mediated by HIF-1α, leading to upregulation of multiple angiogenic factors, including VEGF. Physiological angiogenesis restores oxygen homeostasis, leading to tissue repair. We postulate that physiological angiogenesis is instrumental in plaque regression. Inability to resolve hypoxia characterizes pathological angiogenesis, leading to persistent VEGF upregulation and sustained angiogenic response. Immature neovessel formation leads to IPH, the main mechanism of necrotic core expansion, oxidation, and inflammation in complex atherosclerosis. The defense mechanisms against IPH include the Hp protein, CD163 scavenger receptor, and the HO-1 protein. Accumulating experimental and clinical data suggest that the Hp 2–2 genotype is associated

with increased cardiovascular events in diabetic patients with atherosclerosis.

Specific antiangiogenic therapy resulted in significant reductions in plaque formation and macrophage infiltration in experimental atherosclerosis. Nevertheless, clinical experience with direct anti-VEGF therapy in patients with cancer led to increased cardiovascular events, including hypertension, left ventricular dysfunction, and thrombotic and embolic events. The mechanisms underlying these events include severe endothelial dysfunction, and, more specifically, microvascular rarefaction. Therapeutic approaches at this time are limited to statin therapy, with dramatic changes in lipid composition and neovessel formation in experimental atherosclerosis.

Conflicts of interest

The authors declare no conflicts of interest.

References

1. Fishman, G.I., S.S. Chugh, J.P. Dimarco, *et al.* 2010. Sudden cardiac death prediction and prevention: report from a National Heart, Lung, and Blood Institute and Heart Rhythm Society Workshop. *Circulation* **122:** 2335–2348.
2. Roger, V.L., A.S. Go, D.M. Lloyd-Jones, *et al.* 2012. Executive summary:heart disease and stroke statistics–2012 update: a report from the American Heart Association. *Circulation* **125:** 188–197.
3. Zemplenyi, T., D.W. Crawford & M.A. Cole. 1989. Adaptation to arterial wall hypoxia demonstrated in vivo with oxygen microcathodes. *Atherosclerosis* **76:** 173–179.
4. Fang, S. & P. Salven. 2010. Stem cells in tumor angiogenesis. *J. Mol. Cell. Cardiol.* **50:** 290–295.
5. Potente, M., H. Gerhardt & P. Carmeliet. 2011. Basic and therapeutic aspects of angiogenesis. *Cell* **146:** 873–887.
6. Arroyo, A.G. & M.L. Iruela-Arispe. 2010. Extracellular matrix, inflammation, and the angiogenic response. *Cardiovasc. Res.* **86:** 226–235.
7. Folkman, J. 2007. Angiogenesis: an organizing principle for drug discovery? *Nat. Rev. Drug Discov.* **6:** 273–286.
8. Sluimer, J.C. & M.J. Daemen. 2009. Novel concepts in atherogenesis: angiogenesis and hypoxia in atherosclerosis. *J. Pathol.* **218:** 7–29.
9. Leppanen, O., T. Bjornheden, M. Evaldsson, *et al.* 2006. ATP depletion in macrophages in the core of advanced rabbit atherosclerotic plaques in vivo. *Atherosclerosis* **188:** 323–330.
10. Sluimer, J.C., J.M. Gasc, J.L. van Wanroij, *et al.* 2008. Hypoxia, hypoxia-inducible transcription factor, and macrophages in human atherosclerotic plaques are correlated with intraplaque angiogenesis. *J. Am. Coll. Cardiol.* **51:** 1258–1265.

11. Bahadori, B., E. Uitz, A. Mayer, *et al.* 2010. Polymorphisms of the hypoxia-inducible factor 1 gene and peripheral artery disease. *Vasc. Med.* **15:** 371–374.

12. Carmeliet, P. & R.K. Jain. 2011. Molecular mechanisms and clinical applications of angiogenesis. *Nature* **473:** 298–307.

13. Majmundar, A.J., W.J. Wong & M.C. Simon. 2010. Hypoxia-inducible factors and the response to hypoxic stress. *Mol. Cell.* **40:** 294–309.

14. Semenza, G.L. 2007. Life with oxygen. *Science* **318:** 62–64.

15. Wenger, R.H. & M. Gassmann. 1997. Oxygen(es) and the hypoxia-inducible factor-1. *Biol. Chem.* **378:** 609–616.

16. Mazzone, M., D. Dettori, R. Leite de Oliveira, *et al.* 2009. Heterozygous deficiency of PHD2 restores tumor oxygenation and inhibits metastasis via endothelial normalization. *Cell* **136:** 839–851.

17. Hutter, R., V. Fuster, B. Sauter, C. Valdiviezo, *et al.* 2006. In vitro and in vivo evidence for hypoxia inducible factor 1-alpha expression in macrophages as link between vascular inflammation and angiogenesis. *Circulation* **114:** II 284–II 285.

18. Moreno, P.R., J. Sanz & V. Fuster. 2009. Promoting mechanisms of vascular health: circulating progenitor cells, angiogenesis, and reverse cholesterol transport. *J. Am. Coll. Cardiol.* **53:** 2315–2323.

19. Heistad, D.D., M.L. Armstrong & M.L. Marcus. 1981. Hyperemia of the aortic wall in atherosclerotic monkeys. *Circ. Res.* **48:** 669–675.

20. Moreno, P.R., K.R. Purushothaman, E. Zias, *et al.* 2006. Neovascularization in human atherosclerosis. *Curr. Mol. Med.* **6:** 457–477.

21. Moreno, P.R., K.R. Purushothaman V. Fuster, *et al.* 2002. Intimomedial interface damage and adventitial inflammation is increased beneath disrupted atherosclerosis in the aorta: implications for plaque vulnerability. *Circulation* **105:** 2504–2511.

22. Moreno, P.R., K.R. Purushothaman, V. Fuster, *et al.* 2004. Plaque neovascularization is increased in ruptured atherosclerotic lesions of human aorta: implications for plaque vulnerability. *Circulation* **110:** 2032–2038.

23. Moreno, P.R., K.R. Purushothaman, M. Sirol, *et al.* 2006. Neovascularization in human atherosclerosis. *Circulation* **113:** 2245–2252.

24. Peters, S.A., S. Dogan, R. Meijer, *et al.* 2011. The use of plaque score measurements to assess changes in atherosclerotic plaque burden induced by lipid-lowering therapy over time: the METEOR study. *J. Atheroscler. Thromb.* **18:** 784–795.

25. Nicholls, S.J., C.M. Ballantyne, P.J. Barter, *et al.* 2011. Effect of two intensive statin regimens on progression of coronary disease. *N. Engl. J. Med.* **365:** 2078–2087.

26. Bot, I., J.W. Jukema, I.M. Lankhuizen, *et al.* 2010. Atorvastatin inhibits plaque development and adventitial neovascularization in ApoE deficient mice independent of plasma cholesterol levels. *Atherosclerosis* **214:** 295–300.

27. Nicholls, S.J., J.M. Borgman, S.E. Nissen, *et al.* 2011. Impact of statins on progression of atherosclerosis: rationale and design of SATURN (study of coronary atheroma by intravascular ultrasound: effect of rosuvastatin versus atorvastatin). *Curr. Med. Res. Opin.* **27:** 1119–1129.

28. Feig, J.E., Y. Shang, N. Rotllan, *et al.* 2011. Statins promote the regression of atherosclerosis via activation of the CCR7-dependent emigration pathway in macrophages. *PLoS ONE* **6:** e28534.

29. Tabas, I. 2010 Macrophage death and defective inflammation resolution in atherosclerosis. *Nat. Rev. Immunol.* **10:** 36–46.

30. Williams, K.J., J.E. Feig & E.A. Fisher. 2007. Cellular and molecular mechanisms for rapid regression of atherosclerosis: from bench top to potentially achievable clinical goal. *Curr. Opin. Lipidol.* **18:** 443–450.

31. Williams, K.J., J.E. Feig & E.A. Fisher. 2008. Rapid regression of atherosclerosis: insights from the clinical and experimental literature. *Nat. Clin. Pract. Cardiovasc. Med.* **5:** 91–102.

32. Moore, K.J. & I. Tabas. 2011. Macrophages in the pathogenesis of atherosclerosis. *Cell* **145:** 341–355.

33. Chinetti-Gbaguidi, G., M. Baron, M.A. Bouhlel, *et al.* 2011. Human atherosclerotic plaque alternative macrophages display low cholesterol handling but high phagocytosis because of distinct activities of the PPARgamma and LXRalpha pathways. *Circ. Res.* **108:** 985–995.

34. Potteaux, S., E.L. Gautier, S.B. Hutchison, *et al.* 2011. Suppressed monocyte recruitment drives macrophage removal from atherosclerotic plaques of Apoe-/- mice during disease regression. *J. Clin. Invest.* **121:** 2025–2036.

35. Randolph, G.J. 2011. Immunology. No need to coax monocytes. *Science* **332:** 1268–1269.

36. Chung, A.S., J. Lee & N. Ferrara. 2010. Targeting the tumour vasculature: insights from physiological angiogenesis. *Nat. Rev. Cancer* **10:** 505–514.

37. Folkman, J. & K. Camphausen. 2001. Cancer. What does radiotherapy do to endothelial cells? *Science* **293:** 227–228.

38. Folkman, J. & P. A. D'Amore. 1996. Blood vessel formation: what is its molecular basis? *Cell* **87:** 1153–1155.

39. Purushothaman, K.R., D. Echeverri, V. Fuster, *et al.* 2003. Neovascularization, inflammation and intra-plaque hemorrhage are increased in advanced human atherosclerosis from patients with diabetes mellitus. *Circulation* **108:** 459.

40. Kockx, M.M., C.K.M. Knaapen, M.W. Bosmans, *et al.* 2003. Phagocytosis and macrophage activation associated with hemorrhagic microvessels in human atherosclerosis. *Arterioscler. Thromb. Vasc. Biol.* **23:** 440–446.

41. Kolodgie, F.D., H.K. Gold, A.P. Burke, *et al.* 2003. Intraplaque hemorrhage and progression of coronary atheroma. *N. Engl. J. Med.* **349:** 2316–2325.

42. Nagy, J.A. & D.R. Senger. 2005. VEGF-A, cytoskeletal dynamics, and the pathological vascular phenotype. *Exp. Cell. Res.* **312:** 538–548.

43. Arbustini, E., P. Morbini, A.M. D'Armini, *et al.* 2002. Plaque composition in plexogenic and thromboembolic pulmonary hypertension: the critical role of thrombotic material in pultaceous core formation. *Heart* **88:** 177–182.

44. Takaya, N., C. Yuan, B. Chu, *et al.* 2005. Presence of intraplaque hemorrhage stimulates progression of carotid atherosclerotic plaques: a high-resolution magnetic resonance imaging study. *Circulation* **111:** 2768–2775.

45. Takaya, N., C. Yuan, B. Chu, *et al.* 2006. Association between carotid plaque characteristics and subsequent ischemic cerebrovascular events: a prospective assessment with MRI–initial results. *Stroke* **37:** 818–823.

46. Gutierrez, J., S.W. Ballinger, V.M. Darley-Usmar, *et al.* 2006. Free radicals, mitochondria, and oxidized lipids: the emerging role in signal transduction in vascular cells. *Circ. Res.* **99:** 924–932.

47. Thomas, C., M.M. Mackey, A.A. Diaz, *et al.* 2009. Hydroxyl radical is produced via the Fenton reaction in submitochondrial particles under oxidative stress: implications for diseases associated with iron accumulation. *Redox Rep.* **14:** 102–108.

48. Cutler, R.G. 2005. Oxidative stress profiling: part I. Its potential importance in the optimization of human health. *Ann. N. Y. Acad. Sci.* **1055:** 93–135.

49. Rother, R.P., L. Bell, P. Hillmen, *et al.* 2005. The clinical sequelae of intravascular hemolysis and extracellular plasma hemoglobin: a novel mechanism of human disease. *JAMA* **293:** 1653–1662.

50. Kristiansen, M., J.H. Graverson, C. Jacobson, *et al.* 2001. Identification of hemoglobin scavenger receptor. *Nature* **409:** 198–201.

51. Langlois, M.R. & J.R. Delanghe. 1996. Biological and clinical significance of haptoglobin polymorphism in humans. *Clin. Chem.* **42:** 1589–1600.

52. Melamed-Frank, M., O. Lache, B.I. Enav, *et al.* 2001. Structure-function analysis of the antioxidant properties of haptoglobin. *Blood* **98:** 3693–3698.

53. Guetta, J., M. Strauss, N.S. Levy, *et al.* 2007. Haptoglobin genotype modulates the balance of Th1/Th2 cytokines produced by macrophages exposed to free hemoglobin. *Atherosclerosis* **191:** 48–53.

54. Levy, A.P., J.E. Levy, S. Kalet-Litman, *et al.* 2007. Haptoglobin genotype is a determinant of iron, lipid peroxidation, and macrophage accumulation in the atherosclerotic plaque. *Arterioscler. Thromb. Vasc. Biol.* **27:** 134–140.

55. Asleh, R., S. Marsh, M. Shilkrut, *et al.* 2003. Genetically determined heterogeneity in hemoglobin scavenging and susceptibility to diabetic cardiovascular disease. *Circ. Res.* **92:** 1193–1200.

56. Levy, A.P.A. Roguin, I. Hochberg, *et al.* 2000. Haptoglobin phenotype and vascular complications in patients with diabetes. *N. Engl. J. Med.* **343:** 969–970.

57. Suleiman, M.D. Aronson, R. Asleh, *et al.* 2005. Haptoglobin polymorphism predicts 30-day mortality and heart failure in patients with diabetes and acute myocardial infarction. *Diabetes* **54:** 2802–2806.

58. Levy, A.P., I. Hochberg, K. Jablonski, *et al.* 2002. Haptoglobin phenotype is an independent risk factor for cardiovascular disease in individuals with diabetes: the Strong Heart Study. *J. Am. Coll. Cardiol.* **40:** 1984–1990.

59. Schaer C.A., F. Vallelian, A. Imhof, *et al.* 2007. CD163-expressing monocytes constitute an endotoxin-sensitive Hb clearance compartment within the vascular system. *J. Leucocyte Biol.* **82:** 106–110.

60. Schaer, C.A., G. Schoedon, A. Imhof, *et al.* 2006. Constitutive endocytosis of CD163 mediates hemoglobin-heme uptake and determines the noninflammatory and protective transcriptional response of macrophages to hemoglobin. *Circ. Res.* **99:** 943–950.

61. Schaer, D.J. 2002. The macrophage hemoglobin scavenger receptor CD163 as a genetically determined disease modifying pathway in atherosclerosis. *Atherosclerosis* **163:** 199–201.

62. Philippidis, P., J.C. Mason, B.J. Evans, *et al.* 2004. Hemoglobin scavenger receptor CD163 mediates interleukin-10 release and heme oxygenase-1 synthesis: antiinflammatory monocyte-macrophage responses in vitro, in resolving skin blisters in vivo, and after cardiopulmonary bypass surgery. *Circ. Res.* **94:** 119–126.

63. Schaer, D., F.S. Boretti, A. Hongegger, *et al.* 2001. Molecular cloning and characterization of the mouse CD163 homologue, a highly glucocorticoid-inducible member of the scavenger receptor cysteine-rich family. *Immunogenetics* **53:** 170–177.

64. Siow, R.C., H. Sato, & G.E. Mann. 1999. Heme oxygenase–carbon monoxide signalling pathway in atherosclerosis:antiatherogenic actions of bilirubin and carbon monoxide? *Cardiovasc. Res.* **41:** 385–394.

65. Lin, Q., S. Weis, G. Yang, *et al.* 2007. Heme oxygenase-1 protein localizes to nucleus and activates transcription factors important in oxidative stress. *J. Biol. Chemistry.* **282:** 20621–20633.

66. Hoekstra, K.A., D.V. Godin, J. Kurtu, *et al.* 2003. Heme oxygenase and antioxidant status in cultured aortic endothelial cells isolated from atherosclerosis- susceptible and -resistant Japanese quail. *Mol. Cell. Biochem.* **252:** 253–262.

67. Ahmad, F.K., Z. He & G.L. King. 2005. Molecular targets of diabetic cardiovascular complications. *Curr. Drug Targets.* **6:** 487–494.

68. Meerarani, P., A.P. Levy, K.R. Purushothaman, *et al.* 2008. Down-regulation of Heme oxygenase-1 gene expression is associated with decreased ferritin and increased iron deposition in diabetic atherosclerotic plaques. *Diabetes* **57:** A944–A179.

69. Moreno, P.R. & V. Fuster. 2004. New aspects in the pathogenesis of diabetic atherothrombosis. *J. Am. Coll. Cardiol.* **44:** 2293–2300.

70. Purushothaman, K.R., P. Meerarani, P. Muntner, *et al.* 2011. Inflammation, neovascularization and intra-plaque hemorrhage are associated with increased reparative collagen content: implication for plaque progression in diabetic atherosclerosis. *Vasc. Med.* **16:** 103–108.

71. Lu, M., M. Kuroki, S. Amano, *et al.* 1998. Advanced glycation end products increase retinal vascular endothelial growth factor expression. *J. Clin. Invest.* **101:** 1219–1224.

72. Chala, E., C. Manes, H. Lliades, *et al.* 2006. Insulin resistance, growth factors and cytokine levels in overweight women with breast cancer before and after chemotherapy. *Hormones (Athens).* **5:** 137–146.

73. Hirata, C., K. Nakano, N. Nakamura, *et al.* 1997. Advanced glycation end products induce expression of vascular endothelial growth factor by retinal Muller cells. *Biochem. Biophys. Res. Commun.* **236:** 712–715.

74. Asleh, R., J. Guetta, S. Kalet-Litman, *et al.* 2005. Haptoglobin genotype- and diabetes-dependent differences in iron-mediated oxidative stress in vitro and in vivo. *Circ. Res.* **96:** 435–441.

75. Moreno, P.R., K.R. Purushothaman, P. Meerarani, *et al.* 2008. Haptoglobin genotype is a major determinant of the amount

of iron in the human atherosclerotic plaque. *J. Am. Coll. Cardiol.* **52:** 1049–1051.

76. Moulton, K.S., E. Heller, M.A Konerding, *et al.* 1999. Angiogenesis inhibitors endostatin or TNP-470 reduce intimal neovascularization and plaque growth in apolipoprotein E-deficient mice. *Circulation* **99:** 1726–1732.

77. Crawford, Y. & N. Ferrara. 2009. VEGF inhibition: insights from preclinical and clinical studies. *Cell Tissue Res.* **335:** 261–269.

78. Ferrara, N., K.J. Hillan, H.P. Gerber, *et al.* 2004. Discovery and development of bevacizumab, an anti-VEGF antibody for treating cancer. *Nat. Rev. Drug Discov.* **3:** 391–400.

79. Ryan, A.M., D.B. Eppler, K.E. Hagler, *et al.* 1999. Preclinical safety evaluation of rhuMAbVEGF, an antiangiogenic humanized monoclonal antibody. *Toxicol. Pathol.* **27:** 78–86.

80. Jain, R.K. 2001. Normalizing tumor vasculature with antiangiogenic therapy: a new paradigm for combination therapy. *Nat. Med.* **7:** 987–989.

81. Jain, R.K. 2005. Normalization of tumor vasculature: an emerging concept in antiangiogenic therapy. *Science* **307:** 58–62.

82. Batchelor, T.T., A.G. Sorenson, E. di Tomaso, *et al.* 2007. AZD2171, a pan-VEGF receptor tyrosine kinase inhibitor, normalizes tumor vasculature and alleviates edema in glioblastoma patients. *Cancer Cell* **11:** 83–95.

83. Bottomley, A., C. Coens, F. Efficace, *et al.* 2007. Symptoms and patient-reported well-being: do they predict survival in malignant pleural mesothelioma? A prognostic factor analysis of EORTC-NCIC 08983: randomized phase III study of cisplatin with or without raltitrexed in patients with malignant pleural mesothelioma. *J. Clin. Oncol.* **25:** 5770–5776.

84. Willett, C.G., Y. Boucher, E. di Tomaso, *et al.* 2004. Direct evidence that the VEGF-specific antibody bevacizumab has antivascular effects in human rectal cancer. *Nat. Med.* **10:** 145–147.

85. Willett, C.G., Y. Boucher, D.G. Duda, *et al.* 2005. Surrogate markers for antiangiogenic therapy and dose-limiting toxicities for bevacizumab with radiation and chemotherapy: continued experience of a phase I trial in rectal cancer patients. *J. Clin. Oncol.* **23:** 8136–8139.

86. Winter, P.M., A.M. Neubauer, S.D. Caruthers, *et al.* 2006. Endothelial alpha(v)beta3 integrin-targeted fumagillin nanoparticles inhibit angiogenesis in atherosclerosis. *Arterioscler. Thromb. Vasc. Biol.* **26:** 2103–2109.

87. Vaklavas, C., D. Lenihan, R. Kurzrock, *et al.* 2010 Anti-vascular endothelial growth factor therapies and cardiovascular toxicity: what are the important clinical markers to target? *Oncologist* **15:** 130–141.

88. Gerber, H.P., A.K. Malik, G.P. Solar, *et al.* 2002. VEGF regulates haematopoietic stem cell survival by an internal autocrine loop mechanism. *Nature* **417:** 954–958.

89. Heissig, B., K. Hattori, S. Dias, *et al.* 2002. Recruitment of stem and progenitor cells from the bone marrow niche requires MMP-9 mediated release of kit-ligand. *Cell* **109:** 625–637.

90. Ruzinova, M.B., R.A. Schoer, W. Gerald, *et al.* 2003. Effect of angiogenesis inhibition by Id loss and the contribution of bone-marrow-derived endothelial cells in spontaneous murine tumors. *Cancer Cell* **4:** 277–289.

91. Browder, T.C., E. Butterfield, B.M. Kraling, *et al.* 2000. Antiangiogenic scheduling of chemotherapy improves efficacy against experimental drug-resistant cancer. *Cancer Res.* **60:** 1878–1886.

92. Klement, G., S. Baruchel, J. Rak, *et al.* 2000. Continuous low-dose therapy with vinblastine and VEGF receptor-2 antibody induces sustained tumor regression without overt toxicity. *J. Clin. Invest.* **105:** R15–R24.

93. Sweeney, C.J., K.D. Miller, S.E. Sissons, *et al.* 2001. The antiangiogenic property of docetaxel is synergistic with a recombinant humanized monoclonal antibody against vascular endothelial growth factor or 2-methoxyestradiol but antagonized by endothelial growth factors. *Cancer Res.* **61:** 3369–3372.

94. Jain, R.K., A.V. Finn, F.D. Kolodgie, *et al.* 2007. Antiangiogenic therapy for normalization of atherosclerotic plaque vasculature: a potential strategy for plaque stabilization. *Nat. Clin. Pract. Cardiovasc. Med.* **4:** 491–502.

95. Hausenloy, D.J. & D.M. Yellon. 2008. Targeting residual cardiovascular risk: raising high-density lipoprotein cholesterol levels. *Heart* **94:** 706–714.

96. Rubba, P. 2007. Effects of atorvastatin on the different phases of atherogenesis. *Drugs* **67**(Suppl. 1): 17–27.

97. Wilson, S.H., J. Herrmann, L.O. Lerman, *et al.* 2002. Simvastatin preserves the structure of coronary adventitial vasa vasorum in experimental hypercholesterolemia independent of lipid lowering. *Circulation* **105:** 415–418.

98. Park, H.J., D. Kong, L. Iruela-Arispe, *et al.* 2002. 3-hydroxy-3-methylglutaryl coenzyme A reductase inhibitors interfere with angiogenesis by inhibiting the geranylgeranylation of RhoA. *Circ. Res.* **91:** 143–150.

Ann. N.Y. Acad. Sci. ISSN 0077-8923

ANNALS OF THE NEW YORK ACADEMY OF SCIENCES

Issue: *Evolving Challenges in Promoting Cardiovascular Health*

LDL-cholesterol versus HDL-cholesterol in the atherosclerotic plaque: inflammatory resolution versus thrombotic chaos

Lina Badimon[1,2] and Gemma Vilahur[1]

[1]Cardiovascular Research Center, CSIC-ICCC, Hospital de la Santa Creu i Sant Pau, IIB-Sant Pau and CIBEROBN-Pathophysiology of Obesity and Nutrition, Barcelona, Spain. [2]Cardiovascular Research Chair, Universitat Autònoma de Barcelona, Barcelona, Spain

Address for correspondence: Lina Badimon, Cardiovascular Research Center, c/Sant Antoni MaClaret 167, 08025, Barcelona, Spain. lbadimon@csic-iccc.org

Atherosclerosis is a complex disease in which many processes contribute to lesion development. Yet, it is well accepted that high serum levels of low-density lipoproteins (LDL) play a main role in the initiation and progression of atherosclerosis. Despite currently available optimal LDL-lowering therapies, a worrisome number of clinical events still occur. The protective effect of high-density lipoproteins (HDL) in atherosclerosis, either by suppressing vascular-LDL accumulation, inflammation, oxidation, endothelial damage, and thrombosis, has supported the need of the use of HDL-raising therapies to address this residual risk. Results obtained in some studies, however, have shown that HDL quality, rather than quantity, should be the target of future pharmacological therapies. Here, we will first explore the mechanism by which excess LDL is fundamental in the development of atherosclerosis and its thrombotic complications, behaving as a factor that introduces chaos in the vascular wall. Afterwards, we will explore how functional HDL, through various cellular and molecular mechanisms, facilitates the resolution of this vascular chaos by suppression of atherosclerosis progression and induction of regression.

Keywords: high-density lipoproteins; low-density lipoproteins; atherothrombosis

Introduction

Cardiovascular risk factors

Atherosclerotic vascular disease, which encompasses coronary heart disease, cerebrovascular disease, and peripheral arterial disease, is responsible for the majority of cases of cardiovascular disease (CVD) in both developing and developed countries. Large prospective cohort studies such as the Framingham Heart Study and the Seven Countries Study[1,2] have demonstrated the importance of major CVD risk factors in the appearance of vascular events (Fig. 1). Screening for and treating these conditions has become the basis of many published guidelines of risk assessment and reduction strategies.[3] It is apparent, however, that a substantial proportion of cardiovascular events occur in individuals who exhibit none of these classic risk factors.[4] This has led to an increasing interest in identifying novel biomarkers that might improve the global risk prediction of CVD. In recent years, a number of emerging markers have been proposed as significant predictors of atherosclerosis and its thrombotic complications (Fig. 1). However, the INTERHEART study[5] underscored again the importance of plasma lipoproteins in the pathogenesis of CAD and acute MI. As such, the ApoB:ApoA1 ratio (an index of atherogenic lipoproteins and protective lipoproteins, respectively) appeared as a strong, new risk factor for CVD that highlighted the importance of high-density lipoprotein cholesterol (HDL) levels as a risk-reducing factor. Besides the ApoB:ApoA1 ratio, homocysteine, fibrinogen, lipoprotein(a) [Lp(a)], low-density lipoprotein (LDL) of small dense particle size and high-sensitivity C-reactive protein (hs-CRP) have

doi: 10.1111/j.1749-6632.2012.06480.x

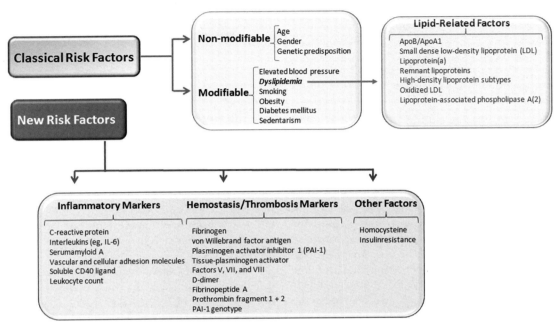

Figure 1. Classical and novel cardiovascular risk factors.

gained interest in the last years to the extent that most of them are accurately measured in routine clinical practice and specific cut-off values have been proposed.[6,7]

LDL and atherosclerosis development

Atherosclerosis: intimal LDL as a triggering factor

Atherosclerosis results from a complex interplay between circulating factors and various cell types in the vessel wall, triggered by the chronic and repeated exposure to pathogenic factors, with high levels of LDL being a key contributor for the initiation and progression of atherosclerosis development.[8–10]

Effect of LDLs on endothelial dysfunction. In healthy conditions, the endothelium controls the vascular tone, maintains the balance between thrombosis and fibrinolysis, and regulates the recruitment of inflammatory cells into the vascular wall. These effects are brought about by the release of several molecules, including nitric oxide (NO), prostacyclin (PGI_2), endothelium-derived hyperpolarizing factor, and endotelin-1. NO plays a central

atheroprotective role through the regulation of vascular tone, inhibition of platelet aggregation, suppression of vascular smooth muscle cell (VSMC) proliferation, and blockade of leukocyte adhesion and transmigration. However, the exposure to high-LDL levels has shown to decrease NO bioavailability either by reducing the concentration and/or activation of NO synthetase (eNOS) or by enhancing NO degradation.[11] Endothelial dysfunction, characterized by the reduction of NO availability, is the preceding step to LDL entry within the arterial intima.

LDL is a heterogeneous class of lipoprotein particles consisting of a hydrophobic core containing triglycerides and cholesterol esters in a hydrophilic shell of phospholipids, free cholesterol, and apolipoproteins, predominantly B-100. The entry and retention of LDL in the subendothelial layer mainly depends on its sustained plasma levels.[12] However, other possible determinants like lipoprotein size, cholesterol enrichment, endothelial permeability, and endothelial cell–derived biosynthetic activity (i.e., synthesis of the basement membrane and extracellular matrix, ECM) may also affect LDL entry and retention.[13]

Once in the intimal space, proteoglycans are responsible for trapping the LDL particles in the arterial intima. Chondroitin sulphate proteoglycans, such as versican, are the main structural proteoglycans of the ECM and are considered important atherogenic elements given that they can strongly interact with, retain, and aggregate cholesterol-rich lipoproteins. LDL particles are those with the greatest capacity for interacting with the proteoglycans. The length and number of glycosaminoglycan chains in proteoglycans produced by VSMCs, as well as their degree of sulfatation, also determines the formation of insoluble complexes between these molecules and the capacity for retention of the LDL particles in the arterial intima. Once retained by ECM components, LDL particles undergo modification processes because of the action of certain oxidants (lipoxygenase, myeloperoxidase, free radicals, etc.) and/or because of proteolytic (kinase, tryptase, metalloproteinases, thrombin, etc.), lipolytic (sphingomyelinase, phospholipase A_2, phospholipase C, etc.), and hydrolytic enzymes (esterase). These chemical and/or structural changes generate different types of modified LDL particles, of which aggregated LDL (agLDL) and oxidated LDL (oxLDL) are the most highly found. In our laboratory, we have demonstrated that the interaction between versican (ECM proteoglycan) and LDL produces structural changes in the LDL particle that lead to agLDL in atherosclerotic lesions.[14,15]

Two families of lipoprotein receptors are considered responsible for LDL uptake by cells of the vascular wall; the LDL receptor family and the scavenger receptor family.

LDL RECEPTOR FAMILY. The first member of the LDL receptor family, the LDL receptor (LDL-R), is involved in the cellular binding and internalization of plasma LDL (native). Other members of this family are the LRP1, LRP-1b and LRP-2/megalin, apolipoprotein E receptor 2 (apoER2), MEGF7, very low-density lipoprotein receptor (VLDL-R), LRP5, and LRP6.[10] Although the LDL-R exclusively mediates the endocytosis of apoE- and apoB- containing lipoprotein particles, LRP1 binds a wide variety of ligands and is involved in multiple internalization processes like endocytosis, phagocytosis, and selective uptake.[16] The LRP1 lipoprotein ligands include apoE-enriched VLDL, lipoprotein lipase, lipoprotein lipase-triglyceride–rich lipoprotein complexes, and Lp(a). In our group, we have identified agLDL

as a new ligand for LRP1.[17] The relevance of LRP1 as a receptor involved on agLDL uptake is enhanced by further demonstration that LRP1 binds and mediates the internalization of agLDL in human coronay and aortic VSMCs, and that this effect is not down-regulated by excess cholesterol, as it is the case for the LDLR. Unlike the LDL-R, which only acts in lipid metabolism, LRP1 also participates in signal transduction. It has been described that LRP1 interacts with the platelet-derived growth factor (PDGF) receptor and that the control of PDGF signaling by LRP1 protects against atherosclerosis.[18] In addition, the cytoplasmic domain of LRP1 has been shown to serve as a docking site for cytoplasmic adaptor and scaffolding proteins involved in signal transduction.[16] Thus, by its dual role as a cargo receptor and a signal transduction receptor, LRP1 regulates critical cellular physiology and signal transduction events.

In macrophages, different pathways for agLDL internalization have been described, among them being pinocytosis, phagocytosis, and pathocytosis. In pathocytosis, agLDL becomes sequestered in large amounts within surface-connected compartments of human monocyte–derived macrophages. LDL uptake into surface-connected compartments has been described to take place through and unidentified receptor.

LRP1 has also been associated with macrophages[19,20] and VSMCs within the human atherosclerotic lesions.[21] Yet, little is known about the factors that regulate LRP1 expression in these cells during atherosclerotic lesion progression. It has been described that LRP1 mRNA levels are increased by colony-stimulating factor-1 and insulin, whereas they are decreased by transforming growth factor-β (TGF-β) and lipopolysaccharide.[10] In our group, we demonstrated that agLDL strongly upregulate LRP1 expression at the transcriptional level, leading to a large increase in LRP1 protein expression.[14] Accordingly, we detected LRP1 over-expression in the vessel wall of hypercholesterolemic animals.[14]

SCAVENGER RECEPTOR FAMILY. The scavenger receptor family has at least eight different subclasses,[22] which bear little sequence homology. Scavenger receptors recognize a wide variety of ligands including oxLDL, apoptotic cells, and pathogens. Although the pathophysiological roles played by these receptors in human disease are still unproven, data from murine models of atherosclerosis have demonstrated a significant role in atherosclerotic foam cell development and vascular lesion development for two receptors, the type A scavenger receptor (SR-A) and the type B scavenger receptor (CD36). SR-A isoforms are largely expressed on macrophages but can also be detected on endothelial and VSMCs.[23] SR-A seems to have a pivotal role on foam cell formation, since mice susceptible to diet-induced atherosclerosis and lacking SR-A showed significantly reduced atherosclerotic lesion size.[24] On the other hand, CD36 is expressed in monocytes, macrophages, platelets, endothelium, adipocytes, and VSMCs. Although SR-A recognizes the oxidized apoprotein portion of the lipoprotein particle, CD36 recognizes lipid moities of oxLDL. Interestingly, CD36 binds with high affinity to a novel class of oxidized phosphatidylcholine found in oxLDL.[10]

Finally, the LOX-1 is a type E scavenger receptor, expressed by endothelial cells, macrophages, and VSMCs, which also recognizes oxLDL. LOX-1 is a type II glycoprotein consisting of a short intracellular domain, a transmembrane-spanning region, and an extracellular C-type lectin domain. In addition to acting as a membrane receptor for oxLDL, soluble forms of LOX-1 have been found to be secreted by TNFα-stimulated endothelial cells.[25]

LDL and innate immunity response in atherosclerosis progression. Another important feature during the development of atherosclerotic lesions is the endothelial transmigration of circulating monocytes into the intravascular space. LDL particles, especially the modified forms, increase the expression and secretion of soluble chemotactic compounds (MCP-1, IL8) and enhance the expression of adhesion molecules such as integrins and selectins, which are exposed on the surface of activated endothelial cells and favor leukocyte (monocyte and T cell) recruitment, adhesion, and transmigration.[9] In addition to the effects on the vascular endothelium, modified LDL particles directly favor the entry of monocytes in the vascular wall through a process that is thought to be mediated by CD11 and the protein kinase C (PKC) pathway. The entry of monocytes takes place through the spaces (junctions) between endothelial cells, preferably in areas where the basal lamina is enriched with modified LDL particles. Then, infiltrated monocytes differentiate into macrophages and express scav-

enger receptors such as CD36 and LOX-1, which internalize many of the cholesterol molecules and cholesterol esters contained in modified LDL particles. Cholesterol internalization leads to the formation of foam cells, a characteristic cell constituent of atherosclerotic lesions. In turn, foam cells secrete proinflammatory cytokines, growth factors, tissue factor (TF), interferon-δ, metalloproteinases (MMP), and reactive oxygen species that maintain the chemotactic stimulus for leukocytes adhered to the vascular endothelium, increase the expression of scavenger receptors, enhance macrophage replication, and regulate VSMC accumulation in the intima.

LDLs and SMC: plaque vulnerability. VSMCs are the major component of the vascular wall that, under the effect of atherogenic stimuli, undergo phenotypic changes ranging from differentiation to the acquisition of a synthetic phenotype. Thus, VSMCs with a nonproliferative contractile phenotype, typical in the vascular media of healthy arteries, transform into actively proliferative cells and migrate toward the vascular intima, attracted by the above-mentioned chemotactic agents.[26] There, VSMCs express a variety of receptors for cholesterol uptake, mainly LRP1, thereby participating in the early accumulation of lipids within the plaque. Although VSMCs account for 90–95% of the cell component in initial lesions, this proportion decreases to 50% in advanced atherosclerotic lesions, making those plaques more vulnerable for rupture. Indeed, unstable plaques contain a substantial lipid core, little collagen, and a small number of VSMCs. These data reflect the importance of identifying and elucidating the cell mechanisms that lead to VSMC loss in advanced lesions. On top of this, atherogenic concentrations of LDL significantly reduce the migratory capacity of human VSMCs, thereby contributing to the vulnerability of these advanced-staged plaques. In this regard, we have recently shown, by proteomic approaches and confocal microscopy, that LDL particles affect the expression and phenotypic profile of different cytoskeleton-related proteins, including the myosin light chain in both the essential and regulatory isoforms.[27] Atherogenic concentrations of LDLs induce myosin regulatory light chain phosphorylation, a key event in the formation of actin–myosin complexes during cell migration and the dynamics of actin fiber formation.[27] This process is highly regulated by proteins such as gelsolin and HSP27.[28]

Impact of LDL on atherothrombosis

Because of the proximity of TF and lipid-rich areas in advanced atherosclerotic lesions, a link between LDL particles, TF expression, and thrombotic risk has been established. Indeed, studies of the relative thrombogenicity of the various components of atherosclerotic plaques have demonstrated that the lipid-rich nucleus is up to six times more thrombogenic than all other components.[29] In addition, we have also shown that inhibition of TF by local administration of TF pathway inhibitor (TFPI) effectively reduces arterial thrombosis in atherosclerotic lesions.[30] TF found in such a lipid-rich core might largely derive from macrophages and VSMC-derived foam cells. Indeed, LDL-laden foam cells have shown to release TF, increasing plaque susceptibility to thrombus formation. On the other hand, we have reported that the interaction between LRP-1 and LDL aggregates is one of the mechanisms that induce VSMC TF expression in a process that depends on RhoA translocation to the membrane and the release of microparticles enriched in active TF to the ECM.[31,32] According to our observations, VSMCs might contribute to increasing not only the thrombogencity of the atherosclerotic plaque but also the circulating TF-enriched microparticles.

LDL levels and the incidence of CVD

Taking in mind the multiple deleterious effects associated with high-LDL cholesterol levels, lipid-lowering strategies have become the cornerstone for the prevention and treatment of CVD. Indeed, the publication of the landmark 4S study showed a total mortality reduction of 29% in ischemic patients treated with simvastatin. Since then, numerous studies have confirmed that statins reduce cardiovascular risk by 20–30%.[33–35] In fact, a recent meta-analysis (14 trials with statins, 90,056 patients, mean follow-up of five years) concluded that for every 40 mg/dL decrease in LDL cholesterol, cardiovascular events are diminished by 21%. These observations suggest the possibility that a more intense LDL-cholesterol reduction could induce higher profits. In fact, this hypothesis was confirmed in several studies using higher doses or more potent statins, such as IDEAL,[36] TNT,[37] and PROVE-IT.[34] Moreover, the ASTEROID study[38] raised the possibility that reducing LDL to an average of 60

mg/dL was associated with a significant regression of atherosclerosis assessed by IVUS after 24 months of treatment. Recently, the SATURN trial has shown that maximal doses of rosuvastatin and atorvastatin resulted in significant regression of coronary atherosclerosis.[39]

Regardless of intensive treatment with statins, the residual risk of having another cardiovascular event remains very high. For instance, despite achieving LDL-C of 62 mg/dL in PROVE-IT,[34] the residual risk of death and ischemic cardiovascular events in patients remained up to 22.4% after two years of follow-up. In other words, alternative strategies are clearly required to bridge the ∼75% gap left after statin treatment in prevention of major cardiovascular events. Efforts are, therefore, currently focused on reducing the residual risk through additional strategies different and complementary to statins, such as increased HDL cholesterol.

Impact of HDL in atherothrombosis

Clinical impact of HDL

Multiple epidemiological studies have provided robust evidence of an inverse correlation between HDL plasma levels and cardiovascular risk.[40] The Framingham study first confirmed that low HDL-cholesterol concentration predicted future cardiovascular events, and was, along with the total cholesterol/HDL, the only independent predictor of CVD. More recent studies (PROCAM,[41] Goldbourt et al.[42]) confirmed this relationship, and found that patients with HDL < 35 mg/dL had an incidence of cardiovascular events eight times higher than individuals with HDL > 65 mg/dL. Moreover, a meta-analysis,[43] including four population studies (FHS,[44] LRCF,[45] CPPT,[46] and MRFIT[47]), showed that for every increase of HDL-cholesterol of 1 mg/dL, there was a 1.9 to 2.3% reduction in cardiovascular risk in men and 3.2% in women. This relationship holds even for low-LDL cholesterol levels. In fact, a post hoc TNT clinical trial, including patients with LDL values below 70 mg/dL, found that those within the highest quintile of HDL-cholesterol had a lower risk of cardiovascular events than those in the lowest quintile.

The importance of HDL was also highlighted in a subanalysis of the MIRACL trial,[48] which showed that low HDL predicts the risk of recurrent cardiovascular events in the short term (four months) after an ACS, while high LDL-C values do not appear to be a prognostic factor. Yet, a recent meta-analysis[49] including four prospective clinical trials that used IVUS (REVERSAL, CAMELOT, ACTI-VATE, ASTEROID) demonstrated that both LDL-C concentrations < 87.5 mg/dL and HDL increase of > 7.5% are simultaneously required to halt plaque progression and achieve plaque regression.

Beneficial effects of HDL in atherothrombosis

It is currently believed that most of the athero-protective effects of HDLs stem from its capacity to remove cholesterol from the vasculature and to deliver it to the liver for disposal in a process commonly referred to as reverse cholesterol transport (RCT). However, during recent years, other features of HDL have been suggested to contribute to its overall anti-atherothrombotic effects, including anti-inflammatory, immunomodulatory, antioxidant, antithrombotic, and endothelial cell repair effects (Fig. 2).[40,50,51]

Reverse cholesterol transport. HDL is a small, dense, spherical lipid-protein structure, with the lipid and protein components each constituting half of the molecule. Major lipid constituents include phospholipid, cholesterol, CE, and triglycerides, whereas the main protein constituents include apoA-1 (constituting approximately 70% of the apolipoprotein content) and apoA-2. Other minor proteins found in smaller amounts include apoC-1, apoC-2, apoC-3, and apo-E.[52] ApoA-1 is produced in the liver and intestine and is initially secreted as a lipid-void apoA-1 molecule, sometimes termed the pre-HDL particle. Lipid components are subsequently added to this particle in the presence of transport proteins such as adenosine triphosphate (ATP)–binding cassette transporter A-1 (ABCA-1). As such, lipid-poor apoA-I interacts with arterial wall macrophage ATP-binding cassette transporter 1 (ABCA1) to remove excess cellular cholesterol from the vessel wall.[53] This lipid-laden ApoA-I becomes the nascent pre-β HDL that starts its remodeling process by esterification of free cholesterol (FC) into CE by lecithin/cholesterol acyltransferase (LCAT) and gets converted into α-HDL. α-HDL may further accept FC from the vessel wall via the SR-B1 receptor present on vessel wall macrophages.[54] The expression of ABCA-1 and SR-B1 is upregulated by excess cellular cholesterol in the form of 27-hydroxycholesterol, which binds to liver X receptor (LXR).[55] LXR, after dimerization with retinoid X receptor (RXR), binds to the LXR promoter and increases expression of both ABCA1 and SR-B1.[56,57] The lipid-laden α-HDL particles deliver CE to the liver via SRB1 or to Apo B–containing lipoproteins, VLDL and LDL, an exchange facilitated by cholesteryl ester transfer protein (CETP).[58] The CE transferred to LDL and VLDL is then targeted for hepatic uptake via LDL receptors (LDLr and LRPr)[59] or accumulates in the arterial wall via subendothelial retention. This mobilization of free cholesterol (RCT) is the principal mechanism behind the benefits associated with elevated HDL, which not only prevents atherosclerosis progression but also offers the possibility to effectively cause regression of established atherosclerotic lesions. In this regard, we demonstrated for the first time in a preclinical animal model the possibility of inducing regression in pre-existent atheroma lesions by HDL-C (HDL3) infusion in a rabbit model of atherosclerosis.[60] At the clinical level, several HDL-raising interventions[38,61] have demonstrated a beneficial effect (reducing atheroma volume) in humans. Some therapies were developed following the observation that certain genetic polymorphisms are associated with high HDL-C levels. Among those that should be highlighted, CETP deficiency and apoA-I mutation, apoA-I Milano, are associated with very high levels of HDL-cholesterol and a very low rate of CVD, respectively. Intravascular ultrasound studies showed, in patients with ACS, that the administration of five weekly intravenous infusions of a reconstituted version of ApoA-I Milano was accompanied by a marked regression of the atherosclerotic plaque, suggesting a very quick and effective RCT.[62] More recently, we have shown by MRI in the atherosclerotic rabbit that only two infusions of apoA-1 Milano are capable of regressing established atherosclerotic lesions,[63] and that this effect is accompanied by an increased plaque stabilization (lower inflammation and apoptosis detection).[63–65] These effects were found less prominent after administration of the native form of apoA-1 than after Apo-A1 Milano.[65,66]

Antioxidant. HDL can also prevent LDL oxidation and scavenge toxic phospholipids from oxidized LDL, thereby protecting VSMCs and endothelial cells. The mechanism behind HDL's antioxidant activity may simply be derived from its high-antioxidant content, but HDL also contains

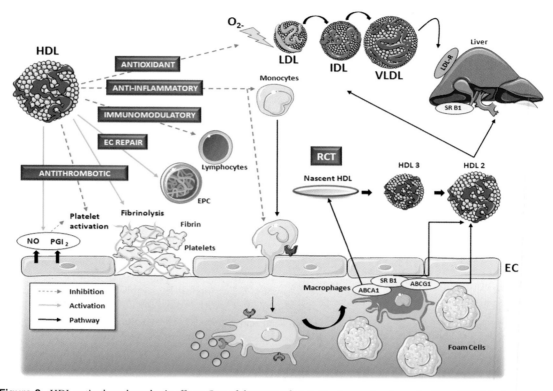

Figure 2. HDL anti-atherothrombotic effects. One of the most atheroprotective mechanisms of action of HDL is the uptake of cholesterol from macrophage-lipid laden cells (foam cells) in the atherosclerosis plaque, after which cholesterol is either transported directly to the liver for excretion into bile or shuttled to LDL/VLDL. This process is termed "reverse cholesterol transport" (RCT). Other important properties of HDL include favorable effects on cell repair (stimulation of endothelial progenitor cell [EPC] recruitment), anti-inflammatory effects (prevention of monocyte attraction/transmigration to the vessel wall), as well as immunomodulatory (modulation of the innate immunity response), antithrombotic (prevention of platelet activation by stimulating nitric oxide [NO] and prostacyclin [PG12] release and stimulating fibrinolysis), and antioxidant (prevention of LDL oxidation) effects.

several antioxidant enzymes that may be involved in degradation of lipid hydroperoxides such as paraoxonase-1 (PON-1), platelet-activating factor acetylhydrolase (PAF-AH), LCAT, and reduced glutathione selenoperoxidase.[67] These antioxidant enzymes may either directly prevent LDL oxidation or degrade oxidized LDL's bioactive products, thereby concomitantly reducing atherosclerosis-related inflammatory response.[67,68] In fact, transgenic animals deficient in PON have shown to be more susceptible to atherosclerosis development,[69] and those that overexpressed PON have less atherosclerosis.[70] Moreover, epidemiologic studies have supported these findings, as high expressor genotypes for PON seem to have a decreased risk of MI,[71] and low PON activity in a cohort of adult men in the Caerphilly Prospective Study[72] was associated with an increased risk of MI.

ApoA-I itself has also shown to exert an antioxidant effect by acting as an acceptor of hydroperoxyeicosatetraenoic acid (HPETE) and hydroperoxydecadienoic acid (HPODE) from native LDL. Both HPETE and HPODE are examples of so-called "seeding molecules," products of 12-lipooxygenase necessary for the induction of nonenzymatic oxidation of LDL phospholipids.[73]

Anti-inflammatory. As detailed above, while the reduction of oxidized LDL may itself result in anti-inflammatory effects, experimental evidence supports that HDL may be directly anti-inflammatory and downregulate endothelial cell adhesion molecules that would otherwise promote monocyte attraction, adhesion, and further migration into the vessel wall.[74] In addition, in a porcine model, HDL has shown to inhibit IL-1α–induced

E-selectin expression by endothelial cells *in vivo* and *ex vivo*, further suggesting HDL-related anti-inflammatory benefits.[75]

Endothelial and vascular function. The mechanism behind HDL's effect on improvement of endothelial function may stem from its antioxidant or anti-inflammatory properties, but HDL may also influence endothelial function independent of these mechanisms as well. Endothelial cells exposed to reconstituted HDL have been observed to have decreased adhesion molecule expression.[76] Furthermore, in hypercholesterolemic men with endothelial dysfunction and in subjects with isolated low HDL, infusion of HDL restored endothelial function by restoring NO bioavailability.[77,78] In fact, NO is increased by apoA1 and sphingosine-1 phosphate (S1P) binding to endothelial SR-B1 and S1P receptors, respectively, and further eNOS activation.[79,80] Furthermore, in our group, we have demonstrated that besides NO, HDL also regulates vascular reactivity through the synthesis of PGI_2 via endothelial cyclooxygenase activation.[81] Interestingly, HDL also regulate vasomotor function by inducing PGI_2 release in human VSMC.[82,83]

Anti-thrombotic. Conflicting results of HDL on platelet activation have been reported. But this is explained by different effects of the various HDL subclasses on platelet activation: HDL3 have been reported to exhibit either no effect on platelets or induces platelet ion-channel activation,[84] whereas inhibition has been reported for HDL2 and apoE-rich HDL.[85] Indeed, HDL2 has shown to reduce thrombin-induced platelet aggregation; 14 C-serotonin release induced by thrombin, ADP, and epinephrine;[85] inhibit platelet shape change and Ca^{2+} mobilization; and reduce eNOS expression induced by oxidized LDL.[86] Inhibition of platelet function by HDL2 is mediated by apoE, since chemical modification of lysine, arginine, and tyrosine residues in apoE of HDL has shown to abolish binding and the antiaggregatory effect. In addition, apoA is also involved in inhibition of platelet functions, albeit to a lesser degree than apoE,[87] and addition of apoA-I Milano has been shown to inhibit arterial thrombus formation in a murine model.[88]

HDL also stabilizes PGI_2, a powerful mediator of thromboresistance at the platelet/vessel wall interface.[82,83,89] Interestingly, we have reported that changes in dietary fatty acids may even modulate HDL potential to induce PGI_2 release from VSMCs.[90] This overall antithrombotic potential of HDL particles has been demonstrated with the Badimon perfusion chamber, in which serum HDL level from hypercholesterolemic men was a significant independent predictor of platelet thrombus formation.[91]

Anticoagulant and fibrinolytic properties of HDL have also been demonstrated in *in vitro* studies. On the one hand, purified HDL significantly enhanced inactivation of coagulation factor Va by activation of protein C and protein S.[92] HDL and apoA-I have also been shown to decrease the procoagulant activity of red blood cells.[93] On the other hand, HDL have shown to contain TFPI activity,[94] and the protein components of HDL, specifically apoA-1 and apoA-2, have been found to activate fibrinolysis.[95]

Inhibition of endothelial apoptosis and stimulation of endothelial repair. Different HDL components have been suggested to mediate the anti-apoptotic capacity of the lipoprotein. ApoA-1 has been implicated in inhibition of endothelial cell apoptosis induced by oxidized LDL, VLDL, and TNF-α, whereas HDL-associated lysosphingolipids have been shown to inhibit endothelial cell apoptosis induced by growth factor depletion by preventing the activation of the mitochondrial-mediated apoptosis pathway and leading to Akt activation, an important anti-apoptotic mediator in endothelial cells.[96]

HDL has been also implicated in the stimulation of endothelial repair processes, which have long been thought of to be only dependent on the proliferation and migration of local adjacent endothelial cells. Several recent studies have clearly suggested that bone marrow–derived endothelial progenitor cells (the so-called EPCs) may promote endothelial repair after vascular injury, contribute to endothelial repair processes in lesion-prone areas of experimental atherosclerosis, and improve endothelial function. In this regard, recent work has suggested that HDL stimulates endothelial repair by both promotion of endothelial cell proliferation or migration (by binding of apoA-I to SR-BI or by binding of sphingosine-1-phosphate to its receptors, S1P1 and S1P3) and/or stimulation of EPC recruitment.[97]

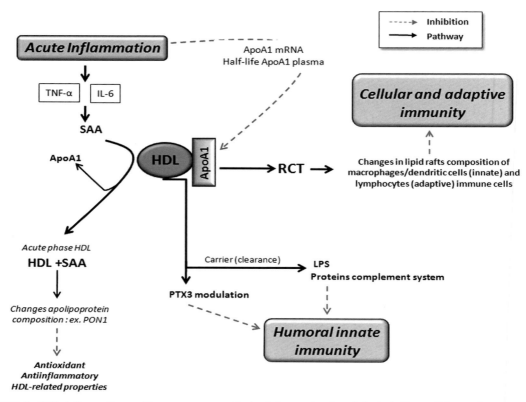

Figure 3. HDL, inflammation, and immune response. During inflammation (e.g., infection), IL-6 and TNFα release stimulate the expression of serum amyloid A (SAA), which dramatically alters HDL apolipoprotein content (replaces ApoA1) and thereby partially impairs HDL-atheroprotective properties. Yet, HDL has also the capacity to tune the inflammatory response and antigen presentation. Indeed, depletion of cholesterol from lipid rafts following HDL interaction modulates the activity and function of cells of the innate and adaptive immune system. Moreover, by acting as carriers of proteins of the complement system and modulating pentraxin -3 (PTX3), HDL also influences the humoral innate immunity.

Acute-phase HDL and immunomodulation. HDL levels have been found altered in several immune-mediated disorders, suggesting an active role of HDL in immunity. Moreover, upon an infection, circulating HDL has showed modified composition and ApoA1 reduction (Fig. 3). In this latter regard, it has been suggested that inflammatory induction of IL-6 and TNF-α induces the expression of serum amyloid A (SAA), which, in turn, displaces ApoA1 for the HDL particle thereby becoming SAA the main HDL protein constituent. These changes in HDL composition (forming the so-called "acute-phase HDL") may alter HDL antiatherogenic potential (e.g., PON1 decrease; Fig. 3). Nevertheless, HDL has also shown the potential to hinder the inflammatory response and antigen presentation functions. In fact, recent data suggest the ability of HDL to modulate both innate and adaptive immune responses

(Fig. 3).[98] HDL, by promoting cholesterol removal (RCT) from immune cell lipid rafts, has been shown to modulate the activity and function of macrophages/denditric cells (innate-) and lymphocytes (adaptive-immune response). Moreover, HDL has also shown to inhibit LPS-induced diffusion and further activation of the innate immune receptor Toll-like receptor (TLR) towards these lipid-rich microdomains. Finally, several studies have also speculated the capacity of HDL to act as a reservoir for biological molecules (LPS and proteins from the complement system), promoting their clearance, and influencing humoral immune response.

Strategies to raise HDL: quality versus quantity?

Several nonpharmacological (life-style related) and pharmacological (monotherapy and/or

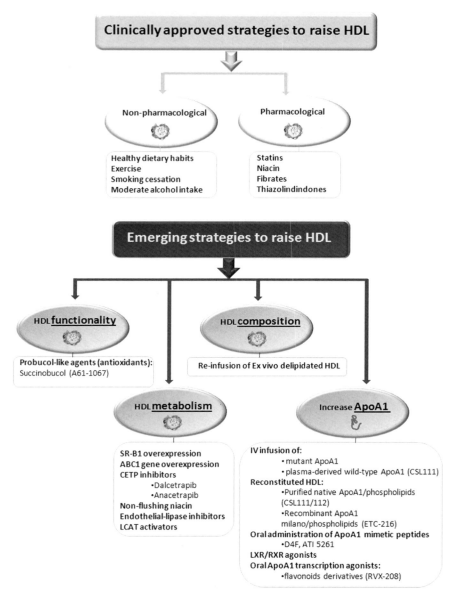

Figure 4. HDL-based therapies. The above depicts the most widely used and clinically proven strategies and cardiovascular drugs to raise HDL (upper panel) as well as promising HDL-raising therapeutics that are under development (lower panel).

combined lipid-modifying therapies) approaches have demonstrated the ability to increase HDL to a varying extent and improve cardiovascular outcomes (Fig. 4).[40,99] However, understanding the biological basis of HDL metabolism has allowed the appearance of new potential therapeutic targets that hold promise for raising HDL as shown in Figure 4. Whether or not any of these drugs and interventions will come to fruition is uncertain; in fact, increasing evidence has introduced the notion that the request for an "HDL drug" should take HDL function into consideration rather than HDL-cholesterol levels increase as the main objective. For instance, for torcetrapib, a CETP inhibitor that was recently being tested in the ILUMINATE trial,[100] despite showing a significant

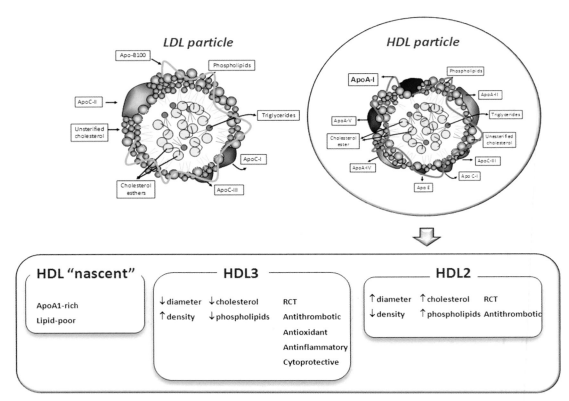

Figure 5. LDL and HDL composition and subtypes. There are three major subtypes of HDL: pre-β (or nascent) HDL, HDL3, and HDL2. As HDL cholesterol is transported, it progresses through these subtypes. The pre-β, or nascent, HDL particle contains very little cholesterol but does contain the major cardioprotective HDL apolipoprotein, apoA-I. Apo A-I in the circulating nascent HDL binds cholesterol, and as it does, it is converted to cholesteryl ester, filling out the nascent HDL so that it changes to a spheroidal particle, HDL3. Eventually, after picking up and transforming more cholesterol to cholesteryl ester, the HDL3 changes in size and density to form the largest HDL particle, HDL2, essentially changing from an unloaded lipid particle to a loaded one. The different HDL subtypes have shown to exert different antiatherosclerotic effects, HDL3 being the most atheroprotective.

increase in HDL-cholesterol levels, the trial was stopped due to increased deaths in the treated arm. The appearance of life-threatening side-effects (increase in blood pressure)[100,101] in the treated arm was hypothesize to cause such negative results; however, the ILUMINATE trial also advised that the search for new drugs cannot be based on raising HDL-cholesterol levels alone.[102] Although it is well known that lipid-poor ApoA-1–HDL binds avidly to macrophages and thereby removing their cholesterol, there is no information on the fate of the spherical, and perhaps dysfunctional, big HDL-cholesterol particles generated by CETP inhibition. This observation supports that the quality of HDL, rather than the quantity, may influence its atheroprotective effects. Indeed, HDL consists of a number of discrete subpopulations that vary in size, density, and composition of lipids and apolipoproteins, suggesting that the capacity of the different HDL particles to exert anti-atherogenic effects may differ (Fig. 5). In effect, the smaller and denser HDL3 subfraction has shown to exert superior anti-inflammatory, anithrombotic, and antioxidant effects than the larger and less-dense HDL2 subfraction. Yet, these protective capacities may not be derived by variations in HDL particle size but by HDL-associated phospholipid content/apoliprotein composition. Detailed HDL proteomic and/or lipidomic analysis (changes in the amount and type of proteins and lipids bound, as well as protein and lipid modifications) may, therefore, provide further new insights into the heterogeneity of HDL composition under various conditions. In fact, dysfunctional HDL has shown to occur in inflammatory/oxidative states. Van Lenten *et al.*[103] demonstrated, in a pioneering study, that acute phase responses in humans may affect HDL anti-inflammatory capacity. As such, HDL isolated from the same subjects before and after cardiac surgery showed that, before cardiac surgery HDL was able to completely inhibit the LDL-induced increase in monocyte transmigration and lipid hydroperoxide formation, whereas 2–3 days after surgery HDL amplified the LDL-induced monocyte transmigration and was less effective in inhibiting lipid hydroperoxide formation. These observations led to hypothesize HDL transformation from an anti-inflammatory towards a proinflammatory particle. Interestingly, the changes in HDL functionality were accompanied by an increase in HDL-associated acute phase reactants (coeruloplasmin and serum amyloid A), whereas the activities of the HDL associated antioxidant enzymes PON and platelet-factor activating acetylhydrolase were reduced in acute phase HDL.[103] Further studies have supported these seminal findings and detected the loss of HDL antiatherosclerotic and anti-inflammatory properties in patients with chronic inflammatory disorders.[97]

Resolution versus chaos

Unopposed effects of excess levels of LDL in the vessel wall lead to the progression of atherosclerosis and to the vascular chaos of plaque rupture and thrombotic vessel closure. The functional effects of the HDL particles counterbalance the deleterious effects of LDL in the vessel wall. HDL particles antagonize many of the cellular and molecular effects of LDL and remove cholesterol from the vessel wall. This damage resolution effect of HDL can to some extent neutralize the chaos inflicted to the wall by excess LDL infiltration.

Opposing the deleterious effects of excess cholesterol accumulation in the vascular wall requires interventions spanning from lifestyle changes to pharmacological treatments. Presently, there are successful strategies to address this issue. In addition, stimulation of the biological protective barrier against the vascular changes induced by LDL can be accomplished by increasing functional HDL particles to reduce residual risk and gain vascular protection.

In a simplified manner, we can summarize by saying that intimal LDL-cholesterol deposits introduce cellular and molecular chaos in the vascular wall that, if unopposed by functionally active HDL, can procure and promote resolution of the chaos by removing and neutralizing the triggering culprit of the cascade of events that eventually leads to ischemic CVD.

Acknowledgments

This work has been supported by PNS SAF2010-16549 (to LB) from the Spanish Ministry of Science and CIBER OBN06 Instituto Carlos-III (to LB). We thank Fundacion Jesus Serra, Barcelona, for their continuous support. GV is a recipient of a grant from the Science and Education Spanish Ministry (RyC-2009-5495, MICINN, Spain).

Conflicts of interest

The authors declare no conflicts of interest.

References

1. Wilson, P.W. *et al.* 1998. Prediction of coronary heart disease using risk factor categories. *Circulation.* **97:** 1837–1847.
2. Keys, A. 1980. Seven Countries: A Multivariate Analysis of Death and Coronary Heart Disease.
3. 2001. Executive Summary of The Third Report of The National Cholesterol Education Program (NCEP) Expert Panel on Detection, Evaluation, And Treatment of High Blood Cholesterol In Adults (Adult Treatment Panel III). *JAMA.* **285:** 2486–2497.
4. Hackam, D.G. & S.S. Anand. 2003. Emerging risk factors for atherosclerotic vascular disease: a critical review of the evidence. *JAMA.* **290:** 932–940.
5. Yusuf, S. *et al.* 2004. Effect of potentially modifiable risk factors associated with myocardial infarction in 52 countries (the INTERHEART study): case-control study. *Lancet.* **364:** 937–952.
6. Kullo, I.J. & C.M. Ballantyne. 2005. Conditional risk factors for atherosclerosis. *Mayo Clin. Proc.* **80:** 219–230.
7. Assmann, G. *et al.* 2005. Implications of emerging risk factors for therapeutic intervention. *Nutr. Metab. Cardiovasc. Dis.* **15:** 373–381.
8. Badimon, L., G. Vilahur & T. Padro. 2009. Lipoproteins, platelets and atherothrombosis. *Rev. Esp. Cardiol.* **62:** 1161–1178.
9. Badimon, L., R.F. Storey & G. Vilahur. 2011. Update on lipids, inflammation and atherothrombosis. *Thromb. Haemost.* **105**(Suppl 1): S34–S42.
10. Badimon, L. *et al.* 2006. Cell biology and lipoproteins in atherosclerosis. *Curr. Mol. Med.* **6:** 439–456.
11. Vidal, F. *et al.* 1998. Atherogenic concentrations of native low-density lipoproteins down-regulate nitric-oxide-synthase mRNA and protein levels in endothelial cells. *Eur. J. Biochem.* **252:** 378–384.

12. Tabas, I., K.J. Williams & J. Boren. 2007. Subendothelial lipoprotein retention as the initiating process in atherosclerosis: update and therapeutic implications. *Circulation.* **116:** 1832–1844.

13. Flood, C. *et al.* 2004. Molecular mechanism for changes in proteoglycan binding on compositional changes of the core and the surface of low-density lipoprotein-containing human apolipoprotein B100. *Arterioscler. Thromb. Vasc. Biol.* **24:** 564–570.

14. Llorente-Cortes, V. *et al.* 2002. Low-density lipoprotein up-regulates low-density lipoprotein receptor-related protein expression in vascular smooth muscle cells: possible involvement of sterol regulatory element binding protein-2-dependent mechanism. *Circulation.* **106:** 3104–3110.

15. Guyton, J.R., K.F. Klemp & M.P. Mims. 1991. Altered ultrastructural morphology of self-aggregated low density lipoproteins: coalescence of lipid domains forming droplets and vesicles. *J. Lipid Res.* **32:** 953–962.

16. Llorente-Cortes, V. & L. Badimon. 2005. LDL receptor-related protein and the vascular wall: implications for atherothrombosis. *Arterioscler. Thromb. Vasc. Biol.* **25:** 497–504.

17. Llorente-Cortes, V., J. Martinez-Gonzalez & L. Badimon. 2000. LDL receptor-related protein mediates uptake of aggregated LDL in human vascular smooth muscle cells. *Arterioscler. Thromb. Vasc. Biol.* **20:** 1572–1579.

18. Boucher, P. *et al.* 2003. LRP: role in vascular wall integrity and protection from atherosclerosis. *Science.* **300:** 329–332.

19. Llorente-Cortes, V. *et al.* 2007. Adipocyte differentiation-related protein is induced by LRP1-mediated aggregated LDL internalization in human vascular smooth muscle cells and macrophages. *J. Lipid. Res.* **48:** 2133–2140.

20. Llorente-Cortes, V. *et al.* 2007. Sterol regulatory element binding proteins downregulate LDL receptor-related protein (LRP1) expression and LRP1-mediated aggregated LDL uptake by human macrophages. *Cardiovasc. Res.* **74:** 526–536.

21. Llorente-Cortes, V. *et al.* 2004. Intracellular lipid accumulation, low-density lipoprotein receptor-related protein expression, and cell survival in vascular smooth muscle cells derived from normal and atherosclerotic human coronaries. *Eur. J. Clin. Invest.* **34:** 182–190.

22. Yla-Herttuala, S. 1999. Oxidized LDL and atherogenesis. *Ann. N. Y. Acad. Sci.* **874:** 134–137.

23. Svensson, L. *et al.* 2002. Inhibitory effects of N-acetylcysteine on scavenger receptor class A expression in human macrophages. *J. Intern. Med.* **251:** 437–446.

24. Kamada, N., T. Kodama & H. Suzuki. 2001. Macrophage scavenger receptor (SR-A I/II) deficiency reduced diet-induced atherosclerosis in C57BL/6J mice. *J. Atheroscler. Thromb.* **8:** 1–6.

25. Murase, T. *et al.* 2000. Identification of soluble forms of lectin-like oxidized LDL receptor-1. *Arterioscler. Thromb. Vasc. Biol.* **20:** 715–720.

26. Doran, A.C., N. Meller & C.A. McNamara. 2008. Role of smooth muscle cells in the initiation and early progression of atherosclerosis. *Arterioscler. Thromb. Vasc. Biol.* **28:** 812–819.

27. Padro, T. *et al.* 2008. Low-density lipoproteins impair migration of human coronary vascular smooth muscle cells and induce changes in the proteomic profile of myosin light chain. *Cardiovasc. Res.* **77:** 211–220.

28. Garcia-Arguinzonis, M. *et al.* Low-density lipoproteins induce heat shock protein 27 dephosphorylation, oligomerization, and subcellular relocalization in human vascular smooth muscle cells. *Arterioscler. Thromb. Vasc. Biol.* **30:** 1212–1219.

29. Fernandez-Ortiz, A. *et al.* 1994. Characterization of the relative thrombogenicity of atherosclerotic plaque components: implications for consequences of plaque rupture. *J. Am. Coll. Cardiol.* **23:** 1562–1569.

30. Badimon, J.J. *et al.* 1999. Local inhibition of tissue factor reduces the thrombogenicity of disrupted human atherosclerotic plaques: effects of tissue factor pathway inhibitor on plaque thrombogenicity under flow conditions. *Circulation.* **99:** 1780–1787.

31. Camino-Lopez, S. *et al.* 2007. Tissue factor induction by aggregated LDL depends on LDL receptor-related protein expression (LRP1) and Rho A translocation in human vascular smooth muscle cells. *Cardiovasc. Res.* **73:** 208–216.

32. Llorente-Cortes, V. *et al.* 2004. Aggregated low-density lipoprotein uptake induces membrane tissue factor procoagulant activity and microparticle release in human vascular smooth muscle cells. *Circulation.* **110:** 452–459.

33. Downs, J.R. *et al.* 1998. Primary prevention of acute coronary events with lovastatin in men and women with average cholesterol levels: results of AFCAPS/TexCAPS. Air Force/Texas Coronary Atherosclerosis Prevention Study. *JAMA.* **279:** 1615–1622.

34. Cannon, C.P. *et al.* 2004. Intensive versus moderate lipid lowering with statins after acute coronary syndromes. *N. Engl. J. Med.* **350:** 1495–1504.

35. 2002. MRC/BHF Heart Protection Study of cholesterol lowering with simvastatin in 20,536 high-risk individuals: a randomised placebo-controlled trial. *Lancet.* **360:** 7–22.

36. Pedersen, T.R. *et al.* 2005. High-dose atorvastatin vs usual-dose simvastatin for secondary prevention after myocardial infarction: the IDEAL study: a randomized controlled trial. *JAMA.* **294:** 2437–2445.

37. LaRosa, J.C. *et al.* 2005. Intensive lipid lowering with atorvastatin in patients with stable coronary disease. *N. Engl. J. Med.* **352:** 1425–1435.

38. Nissen, S.E. *et al.* 2006. Effect of very high-intensity statin therapy on regression of coronary atherosclerosis: the ASTEROID trial. *JAMA.* **295:** 1556–1565.

39. Nicholls, S.J. *et al.* Effect of two intensive statin regimens on progression of coronary disease. *N. Engl. J. Med.* **365:** 2078–2087.

40. Badimon, J.J., C.G. Santos-Gallego & L. Badimon. [Importance of HDL cholesterol in atherothrombosis: how did we get here? Where are we going?]. *Rev. Esp. Cardiol.* **63**(Suppl 2): 20–35.

41. Assmann, G. *et al.* 1996. High-density lipoprotein cholesterol as a predictor of coronary heart disease risk. The PROCAM experience and pathophysiological implications for

reverse cholesterol transport. *Atherosclerosis.* **124**(Suppl): S11–20.

42. Goldbourt, U., S. Yaari & J.H. Medalie. 1997. Isolated low HDL cholesterol as a risk factor for coronary heart disease mortality. A 21-year follow-up of 8000 men. *Arterioscler. Thromb. Vasc. Biol.* **17:** 107–113.

43. Gordon, D.J. *et al.* 1989. High-density lipoprotein cholesterol and cardiovascular disease. Four prospective American studies. *Circulation.* **79:** 8–15.

44. Gordon, T. *et al.* 1977. High density lipoprotein as a protective factor against coronary heart disease. The Framingham Study. *Am J Med.* **62:** 707–714.

45. 1979. Plasma lipid distributions in selected North American populations: the Lipid Research Clinics Program Prevalence Study. The Lipid Research Clinics Program Epidemiology Committee. *Circulation.* **60:** 427–439.

46. 1984. Lipid Research Clinics Program. *JAMA.* **252:** 2545–2548.

47. 1982. Multiple risk factor intervention trial. Risk factor changes and mortality results. Multiple Risk Factor Intervention Trial Research Group. *JAMA.* **248:** 1465–1477.

48. Olsson, A.G. *et al.* 2005. High-density lipoprotein, but not low-density lipoprotein cholesterol levels influence short-term prognosis after acute coronary syndrome: results from the MIRACL trial. *Eur. Heart. J.* **26:** 890–896.

49. Nicholls, S.J. *et al.* 2007. Statins, high-density lipoprotein cholesterol, and regression of coronary atherosclerosis. *JAMA.* **297:** 499–508.

50. Ibanez, B., G. Vilahur & J.J. Badimon. 2007. Plaque progression and regression in atherothrombosis. *J. Thromb. Haemost.* **5**(Suppl 1): 292–299.

51. Choi, B.G. *et al.* 2006. The role of high-density lipoprotein cholesterol in atherothrombosis. *Mt. Sinai. J. Med.* **73:** 690–701.

52. Singh, V. *et al.* Low high-density lipoprotein cholesterol: current status and future strategies for management. *Vasc. Health. Risk. Manag.* **6:** 979–996.

53. Liu, L. *et al.* 2003. Effects of apolipoprotein A-I on ATP-binding cassette transporter A1-mediated efflux of macrophage phospholipid and cholesterol: formation of nascent high density lipoprotein particles. *J Biol. Chem.* **278:** 42976–42984.

54. Williams, D.L. *et al.* 1999. Scavenger receptor BI and cholesterol trafficking. *Curr. Opin. Lipidol.* **10:** 329–339.

55. Fu, X. *et al.* 2001. 27-hydroxycholesterol is an endogenous ligand for liver X receptor in cholesterol-loaded cells. *J. Biol. Chem.* **276:** 38378–38387.

56. Malerod, L. *et al.* 2002. Oxysterol-activated LXRalpha/RXR induces hSR-BI-promoter activity in hepatoma cells and preadipocytes. *Biochem. Biophys. Res. Commun.* **299:** 916–923.

57. Venkateswaran, A. *et al.* 2000. Control of cellular cholesterol efflux by the nuclear oxysterol receptor LXR alpha. *Proc. Natl. Acad. Sci. U S A.* **97:** 12097–12102.

58. Trigatti, B.L., M. Krieger & A. Rigotti. 2003. Influence of the HDL receptor SR-BI on lipoprotein metabolism and atherosclerosis. *Arterioscler. Thromb. Vasc. Biol.* **23:** 1732–1738.

59. Goldstein, J.L. & M.S. Brown. 1987. Regulation of low-density lipoprotein receptors: implications for pathogenesis and therapy of hypercholesterolemia and atherosclerosis. *Circulation.* **76:** 504–507.

60. Badimon, J.J. *et al.* 1989. High density lipoprotein plasma fractions inhibit aortic fatty streaks in cholesterol-fed rabbits. *Lab. Invest.* **60:** 455–461.

61. Taylor, A.J., H.J. Lee & L.E. Sullenberger. 2006. The effect of 24 months of combination statin and extended-release niacin on carotid intima-media thickness: ARBITER 3. *Curr. Med. Res. Opin.* **22:** 2243–2250.

62. Nissen, S.E. *et al.* 2003. Effect of recombinant ApoA-I Milano on coronary atherosclerosis in patients with acute coronary syndromes: a randomized controlled trial. *JAMA.* **290:** 2292–2300.

63. Ibanez, B. *et al.* 2008. Rapid change in plaque size, composition, and molecular footprint after recombinant apolipoprotein A-I Milano (ETC-216) administration: magnetic resonance imaging study in an experimental model of atherosclerosis. *J. Am. Coll. Cardiol.* **51:** 1104–1109.

64. Cimmino, G. *et al.* 2009. Up-regulation of reverse cholesterol transport key players and rescue from global inflammation by ApoA-I(Milano). *J. Cell. Mol. Med.* **13:** 3226–3235.

65. Ibanez, B. *et al.* 2012. Recombinant HDL(Milano) exerts greater anti-inflammatory and plaque stabilizing properties than HDL(wild-type). *Atherosclerosis* **220:** 72–77.

66. Cimmino, G. *et al.* 2009. Up-regulation of reverse cholesterol transport key players and rescue from global inflammation by ApoA-I. *J. Cell. Mol. Med.* **13:** 3226–3235.

67. Navab, M. *et al.* 2001. HDL and the inflammatory response induced by LDL-derived oxidized phospholipids. *Arterioscler. Thromb. Vasc. Biol.* **21:** 481–488.

68. Aviram, M. *et al.* 2000. Human serum paraoxonases (PON1) Q and R selectively decrease lipid peroxides in human coronary and carotid atherosclerotic lesions: PON1 esterase and peroxidase-like activities. *Circulation.* **101:** 2510–2517.

69. Shih, D.M. *et al.* 1998. Mice lacking serum paraoxonase are susceptible to organophosphate toxicity and atherosclerosis. *Nature.* **394:** 284–287.

70. Tward, A. *et al.* 2002. Decreased atherosclerotic lesion formation in human serum paraoxonase transgenic mice. *Circulation.* **106:** 484–490.

71. Leviev, I. *et al.* 2002. High expressor paraoxonase PON1 gene promoter polymorphisms are associated with reduced risk of vascular disease in younger coronary patients. *Atherosclerosis.* **161:** 463–467.

72. Mackness, B. *et al.* 2003. Low paraoxonase activity predicts coronary events in the Caerphilly Prospective Study. *Circulation.* **107:** 2775–2779.

73. Assmann, G. & A.M. Gotto, Jr. 2004. HDL cholesterol and protective factors in atherosclerosis. *Circulation.* **109:** III8–14.

74. Barter, P.J., P.W. Baker & K.A. Rye. 2002. Effect of high-density lipoproteins on the expression of adhesion molecules in endothelial cells. *Curr. Opin. Lipidol.* **13:** 285–288.

75. Cockerill, G.W. *et al.* 2001. Elevation of plasma high-density lipoprotein concentration reduces interleukin-1-induced expression of E-selectin in an in vivo model of acute inflammation. *Circulation.* **103**: 108–112.

76. Clay, M.A. *et al.* 2001. Time sequence of the inhibition of endothelial adhesion molecule expression by reconstituted high density lipoproteins. *Atherosclerosis.* **157**: 23–29.

77. Spieker, L.E. *et al.* 2002. High-density lipoprotein restores endothelial function in hypercholesterolemic men. *Circulation.* **105**: 1399–1402.

78. Bisoendial, R.J. *et al.* 2003. Restoration of endothelial function by increasing high-density lipoprotein in subjects with isolated low high-density lipoprotein. *Circulation.* **107**: 2944–2948.

79. Rodriguez, C. *et al.* 2009. Sphingosine-1-phosphate: a bioactive lipid that confers high-density lipoprotein with vasculoprotection mediated by nitric oxide and prostacyclin. *Thromb. Haemost.* **101**: 665–673.

80. Yuhanna, I.S. *et al.* 2001. High-density lipoprotein binding to scavenger receptor-BI activates endothelial nitric oxide synthase. *Nat. Med.* **7**: 853–857.

81. Gonzalez-Diez, M. *et al.* 2008. Prostacyclin induction by high-density lipoprotein (HDL) in vascular smooth muscle cells depends on sphingosine 1-phosphate receptors: effect of simvastatin. *Thromb. Haemost.* **100**: 119–126.

82. Vinals, M. *et al.* 1997. HDL-induced prostacyclin release in smooth muscle cells is dependent on cyclooxygenase-2 (Cox-2). *Arterioscler. Thromb. Vasc. Biol.* **17**: 3481–3488.

83. Vinals, M., J. Martinez-Gonzalez & L. Badimon. 1999. Regulatory effects of HDL on smooth muscle cell prostacyclin release. *Arterioscler. Thromb. Vasc. Biol.* **19**: 2405–2411.

84. Nofer, J.R. *et al.* 1996. High density lipoproteins enhance the Na+/H+ antiport in human platelets. *Thromb. Haemost.* **75**: 635–641.

85. Aviram, M. *et al.* 1985. Plasma lipoproteins affect platelet malondialdehyde and thromboxane B2 production. *Biochem. Med.* **34**: 29–36.

86. Mehta, J.L. & L.Y. Chen. 1996. Reversal by high-density lipoprotein of the effect of oxidized low-density lipoprotein on nitric oxide synthase protein expression in human platelets. *J. Lab. Clin. Med.* **127**: 287–295.

87. Korporaal, S.J. & J.W. Akkerman. 2006. Platelet activation by low density lipoprotein and high density lipoprotein. *Pathophysiol. Haemost. Thromb.* **35**: 270–280.

88. Li, D. *et al.* 1999. Inhibition of arterial thrombus formation by ApoA1 Milano. *Arterioscler. Thromb. Vasc. Biol.* **19**: 378–383.

89. Pirich, C. *et al.* 1997. Hyperalphalipoproteinemia and prostaglandin I2 stability. *Thromb. Res.* **88**: 41–49.

90. Escudero, I. *et al.* 2003. Experimental and interventional dietary study in humans on the role of HDL fatty acid composition in PGI2 release and Cox-2 expression by VSMC. *Eur. J. Clin. Invest.* **33**: 779–786.

91. Naqvi, T.Z. *et al.* 1999. Evidence that high-density lipoprotein cholesterol is an independent predictor of acute platelet-dependent thrombus formation. *Am. J. Cardiol.* **84**: 1011–1017.

92. Griffin, J.H. *et al.* 1999. High-density lipoprotein enhancement of anticoagulant activities of plasma protein S and activated protein C. *J. Clin. Invest.* **103**: 219–227.

93. Epand, R.M. *et al.* 1994. HDL and apolipoprotein A-I protect erythrocytes against the generation of procoagulant activity. *Arterioscler. Thromb.* **14**: 1775–1783.

94. Lesnik, P. *et al.* 1993. Anticoagulant activity of tissue factor pathway inhibitor in human plasma is preferentially associated with dense subspecies of LDL and HDL and with Lp(a). *Arterioscler. Thromb.* **13**: 1066–1075.

95. Saku, K. *et al.* 1985. Activation of fibrinolysis by apolipoproteins of high density lipoproteins in man. *Thromb. Res.* **39**: 1–8.

96. Nofer, J.R. *et al.* 2001. Suppression of endothelial cell apoptosis by high density lipoproteins (HDL) and HDL-associated lysosphingolipids. *J. Biol. Chem.* **276**: 34480–34485.

97. Besler, C. *et al.* High-density lipoprotein-mediated anti-atherosclerotic and endothelial-protective effects: a potential novel therapeutic target in cardiovascular disease. *Curr. Pharm. Des.* **16**: 1480–1493.

98. Norata, G.D. *et al.* Emerging role of high density lipoproteins as a player in the immune system. *Atherosclerosis.* **220**: 11–21.

99. Choi, B.G. *et al.* 2006. The role of high-density lipoprotein cholesterol in the prevention and possible treatment of cardiovascular diseases. *Curr. Mol. Med.* **6**: 571–587.

100. Barter, P.J. *et al.* 2007. Effects of torcetrapib in patients at high risk for coronary events. *N. Engl. J. Med.* **357**: 2109–2122.

101. Blasi, E. *et al.* 2009. Effects of CP-532,623 and torcetrapib, cholesteryl ester transfer protein inhibitors, on arterial blood pressure. *J. Cardiovasc. Pharmacol.* **53**: 507–516.

102. Barter, P. 2009. Lessons learned from the Investigation of Lipid Level Management to Understand its Impact in Atherosclerotic Events (ILLUMINATE) trial. *Am. J. Cardiol.* **104**: 10E–15E.

103. Van Lenten, B.J. *et al.* 1995. Anti-inflammatory HDL becomes pro-inflammatory during the acute phase response. Loss of protective effect of HDL against LDL oxidation in aortic wall cell cocultures. *J. Clin. Invest.* **96**: 2758–2767.

Ann. N.Y. Acad. Sci. ISSN 0077-8923

ANNALS OF THE NEW YORK ACADEMY OF SCIENCES
Issue: *Evolving Challenges in Promoting Cardiovascular Health*

Evolving role of molecular imaging for new understanding: targeting myofibroblasts to predict remodeling

Hans J. de Haas,[1,2,*] Susanne W. van den Borne,[3,*] Hendrikus H. Boersma,[2,4] Riemer H.J.A. Slart,[2] Valentin Fuster,[1,5] and Jagat Narula[1]

[1]Zena and Michael A. Wiener Cardiovascular Institute, Mount Sinai School of Medicine, New York, New York. [2]Department of Nuclear Medicine and Molecular Imaging, Cardiovascular Imaging Group Groningen, University Medical Center Groningen, University of Groningen, the Netherlands. [3]Department of Gynecology and Obstetrics, Maastricht University Medical Center, Maastricht, the Netherlands. [4]Department of Clinical and Hospital Pharmacy, University Medical Center Groningen, University of Groningen, Groningen, the Netherlands. [5]Centro Nacional de Investigaciones Cardiovasculares (CNIC), Madrid, Spain

Address for correspondence: Jagat Narula, M.D./Ph.D., Zena and Michael A. Wiener Cardiovascular Institute, Mount Sinai School of Medicine, New York, NY 10029. narula@mountsinai.org

Containment of the process of cardiac remodeling is a prerequisite for prevention of development of heart failure (HF) after myocardial infarction. For personalization of therapeutic intervention strategy, it may be of benefit to identify the subset of patients who are at higher risk for development of HF. One such strategy may involve targeted imaging of various components involved in the remodeling process and interstitial fibrosis, including the myofibroblast. This cell type combines characteristics of fibroblasts and smooth muscle cells, and plays a crucial role in infarct healing and scar contraction. We define molecular targets on myofibroblasts and discuss the feasibility of molecular imaging of these cells for early detection and treatment of patients at risk for development of HF after myocardial infarction.

Keywords: myocardial infarction; adverse remodeling; heart failure; molecular imaging; fibrosis; myofibroblast

Introduction

In the immediate aftermath of myocardial infarction (MI), the healing process is initiated. In this process, three overlapping phases are recognized; inflammatory, proliferatory, and the maturation phase.[1,2] Inflammatory cells infiltrate into the infarct area and contribute to removal of the cellular debris. After approximately four days, granulomatous tissue comprising myofibroblasts and newly formed vessels develops within the infarct area. A variety of growth factors and neurohormones, such as vascular endothelial growth factor (VEGF), fibroblast growth factor (FGF), platelet-derived growth factor (PDGF), angiotensin II, and transforming growth factor β (TGF-β), are implicated in this process. TGF-β is has been deemed responsible for the activation and proliferation of fibroblasts

within the heart and triggers their differentiation into myofibroblasts.[3] TGF-β may also cause transdifferentiation of endothelial and epithelial cells into myofibroblasts.[4] TGF-signaling is further stimulated by angiotensin II, which is upregulated after MI in macrophages, myofibroblasts, and cardiomyocytes, causing an increased production of angiotensin converting enzyme (ACE) by cardiomyocytes in the infarct border and myofibroblasts within the infarct.[5] When angiotensin II binds to the receptors on myofibroblasts, they produce TGF-β at a higher rate.[5]

Activated myofibroblasts lay down collagen fibers, mostly collagen types I and III, in extracellular matrix.[6] In response to hypoxic signals from the metabolically highly active myofibroblasts, angiogenic vessels are formed to compensate for the ischemic loss of microvasculature and supply the myofibroblasts with nutrients. Concurrent with the proliferation, myofibroblasts produce lysyl oxidase enzymes, that strengthen the collagen network by

---

*Authors contributed equally to the manuscript.

doi: 10.1111/j.1749-6632.2012.06476.x

crosslinking the fibers.[7] In addition, myofibroblasts, which are connected to the collagen microfibers, contract.[8] Although scar formation and contraction contribute to the preservation of pump function, excessive fibrosis both within and outside of the infarct area directly contributes to myocardial remodeling. TGF-β produced in the infarct area may permeate to the spared myocardium and result in accumulation of the activated myofibroblasts.[9] Angiotensin II contributes to accumulation of myofibroblasts.[6] The resulting formation of fibrous tissue in the otherwise healthy areas of the heart results in increased stiffening and systolic and diastolic dysfunction of the heart. Furthermore, the activity of myofibroblasts has been shown to directly influence cardiomyocyte hypertrophy in initially spared myocardium.[10]

Because of the critical role of myofibroblasts in myocardial remodeling, they present the most promising target for a molecular imaging strategy to identify patients at risk for the development of heart failure (HF). In these patients, it is expected that the spread and the density of the myofibroblasts in the infarct and surrounding region, regardless of the restoration of perfusion status, would determine the eventual size and quality of scar and infarct expansion. On the other hand, an excessive number of myofibroblasts in the initially uninjured parts of the heart, would determine interstitial fibrosis and remodeling within the noninfarcted myocardium. In this review, we define potential imaging targets of the myofibroblast, and we describe feasibility of myofibroblast imaging techniques and how these have increased understanding of the pathology and treatment of myocardial adverse remodeling.

Molecular targets in myofibroblasts amenable to imaging

For development of useful imaging techniques within this context, it would be desirable to define moieties that are exclusively expressed by myofibroblasts. Although myofibroblasts express several markers (see Fig. 1), both intracellularly and extracellularly, unfortunately none of these targets are sufficiently exclusive to be highly specific for myofibroblasts.[11]

Myofibroblasts share the expression of α-smooth muscle actin (ASMA) with SMC, which is an early differentiation marker of vascular SMC. Unlike

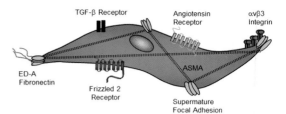

Figure 1. Potential targets for myofibroblast imaging. Myofibroblasts express a variety of molecules that could be used as targets for molecular imaging approaches. Proof of principle studies have shown feasibility of targeting membrane-bound angiotensin receptors and $\alpha_v\beta_3$ integrins. Frizzled-2 receptor and TGF-β receptors could also present promising targets on the cell membrane. ED-A fibronectin and nascent collagen fibers could be used as targets to show myofibroblast activity indirectly. TGF-β: transforming growth factor β.

SMC however, myofibroblasts express relatively low amounts of smooth muscle myosin heavy chain and do not express smoothelin, a late differentiation marker.[12] On the other hand, expression of various (trans) membrane moieties on myofibroblasts may present better targets. The migration and differentiation of myofibroblasts are partially determined by a tissue polarity gene, frizzled 2,[13] which is upregulated in the myofibroblasts during their migration into the infarct area. Because frizzled-2 receptors are located on the plasma membrane they should be easily accessible, provided that specific ligands would be available.

Myofibroblasts also express renin, ACE, ACE-like enzymes, and angiotensin II as well as angiotensin receptors.[5] Increased stimulation by angiotensin II perpetuates collagen synthesis by induction of TGF-β1 expression, which is abrogated by AT1R antagonists. An ongoing expression of angiotensin II and AT1R and active TGF-β1 and TGF-β1 receptors is observed in the infarcted rodent heart for months after MI and underscores persistent metabolic activity of activated myofibroblasts.[5] Angiotensin II, produced locally by activated macrophages, cardiomyocytes, and myofibroblasts, exerts its effect by directly inducing NADPH oxidase activity in myofibroblasts, stimulating TGF-β1 production, and triggering fibroblast proliferation and differentiation into collagen-secreting myofibroblasts. Because of the persistent expression of AT1R on myofibroblasts, they could serve as a suitable target for molecular imaging.

TGF-β1 augments production of interstitial collagens, fibronectin, and proteoglycans by cardiac myofibroblasts. It also perpetuates its own production within myofibroblasts, thereby establishing an autocrine cycle of myofibroblastic differentiation and activation.[14] Studies have shown that overexpression of TGF-β1 in transgenic mice can lead to cardiac hypertrophy, characterized by both interstitial fibrosis and hypertrophic growth of cardiac myocytes.[10] Therefore, TGF-β1 receptors could be another potential target for molecular imaging of myofibroblasts. However, the components of the renin–angiotensin system (RAS) and TGF-β1 signaling, although expressed at high levels on myofibroblasts, are also expressed on other cells and imaging may lack specificity.

Analysis of myofibroblasts in fibrotic and granulation tissue reveals extensive cell-matrix contacts called fibronexi, which are not observed in fibroblasts isolated from normal connective tissue. Cultured myofibroblasts develop specialized focal adhesions (FA) that have been termed supermature FA to account for their significantly longer appearance compared with classical FA of ASMA-negative fibroblasts. In addition, supermature FA exhibit a specific molecular composition by coexpressing high levels of vinculin, paxillin, tensin, and the integrins $\alpha_v\beta_3$ and $\alpha_5\beta_1$.[15] In general, $\alpha_v\beta_3$ integrin expression in myocardium is rare in adults, but it is seen on endothelial cells during angiogenesis in response to angiogenic growth factors, such as basic fibroblast growth factor (bFGF), and is fundamental for endothelial cell proliferation, adhesion, and survival. Because neoangiogenesis and myofibroblastic proliferation occur together in post-MI remodeling, integrin targeting may be a reasonable approach for molecular imaging.

In addition to relatively exclusive membrane markers, it may also be prudent to target the company myofibroblasts keep. In the infarct area, for instance, the presence of myofibroblasts leads to collagen deposition, and collagen crosslinking is mediated by lysyl oxidase family enzymes.[7] Lysyl oxidase is upregulated during the first weeks of infarct healing and remains elevated up to 90 days after MI;[7] its expression is responsive to connective tissue growth factor and TGF-β,[16] and could probably be used as a surrogate marker for the extent of myofibroblast proliferation.

Imaging of upregulation of growth factor receptors on myofibroblasts

As discussed earlier, myocardial upregulation of the RAS system contributes prominently to ventricular remodeling. Myocardial angiotensin II type 1 (AT1R) receptor overexpression is associated with interstitial fibrosis,[17] and AT1R receptor deficient transgenic mice exhibit minimal fibrosis after MI.[18] Angiotensin receptor blockers in MI restrict ventricular remodeling, and reduce morbidity and mortality after MI, regardless of the extent of LV functional deterioration.[19–23] It is therefore conceivable that a diagnostic strategy targeted at detecting the extent of myocardial angiotensin receptor expression would allow identification of patients at risk of developing HF, and optimization of pharmacologic therapy in HF patients. For this purpose, employing molecular imaging techniques, angiotensin was labeled with a fluorescent tracer, which targeted both angiotensin type 1 and 2 receptors with high affinity ($K_i = 3$ pM). Intravital fluorescence microscopy was performed to determine the myocardial upregulation of angiotensin receptors in a murine MI model. After intravital microscopy, pathological characterization of tracer uptake localization was performed using confocal and 2-photon microscopy. To more specifically target type 1 receptors, radionuclide imaging with Technetium-99m (Tc-99m)-labeled losartan, an angiotensin type 1 receptor blocker, was performed using microSPECT/CT.[24] Angiotensin receptor imaging was performed in a large number of mice at various time points after permanent coronary artery ligation and in control animals. No tracer uptake was observed in control animals or in infarct region until the first day after MI. Distinct uptake occurred in the infarct area at 1–12 weeks after MI, with maximum uptake between one week and three weeks; uptake markedly was resolved by 12 weeks after MI. Premortem echocardiographic characterization confirmed left ventricular remodeling and pathologic characterization revealed localization of the tracer with collagen-producing myofibroblasts, and colocalization with ASMA. Radiolabeled losartan uptake in the infarct region was 2.5-fold higher than the control animals. This study demonstrated the feasibility of *in vivo* imaging through targeting of neurohumoral upregulation in the myocardium.

Similar to the angiotensin receptor upregulation, ACE upregulation has also been evaluated by an F-18 labeled ACE-inhibitor, fluoro-benzoyl lisinopril.[25] For this purpose, short-axis myocardial slices explanted from cardiac allograft recipients with end-stage ischemic cardiomyopathy were incubated with the radiotracer. There was specific binding of radiotracer to ACE, which was expressed as luminescence/mm,[2] and was highest in infarct border zone, followed by infarct and remote segments. In slides preincubated with cold lisinopril, uptake reduced to half, demonstrating specificity of the radiotracer. The feasibility of noninvasive imaging with benzoyl-lisonopril has recently been demonstrated.[26] The targeting studies demonstrated that ACE (and probably angiotensin II) upregulation may induce the proliferation of myofibroblasts, which have increased angiotensin receptor density and contribute to collagen deposition. However, it remains to be seen whether imaging targeted to angiotensin receptors and/or ACE will result in a clinically robust imaging strategy.

Imaging of surface moieties of myofibroblasts in the infarct area

Integrin moieties expressed on myofibroblasts enhance promoter activity of collagen genes and reduce metalloproteinase genes. This effect is reversible by abrogation of autocrine TGF-β signaling.[27] The arginine–glycine–aspartic acid (RGD) probes that bind to integrins such as $\alpha_v\beta_3$ have been used to identify myofibroblastic proliferation in postinfarct animal models[28,29] as well as in clinical studies.[30] It has been proposed that the uptake of RGD probe indirectly represents the rate of fibrogenesis or collagen deposition. The first animal study demonstrating myofibroblasts by integrin targeting used Cy5.5-RGD imaging peptide (CRIP) labeled with Tc-99m in a murine model of ventricular dysfunction after MI.[28] The fluorescent moiety of the targeting peptide was exploited for immuno-electron microscopic characterization of the probe localization. Again, MI was induced in Swiss-Webster mice by coronary artery occlusion for imaging 2, 4, and 12 weeks after MI. MicroSPECT/CT imaging was performed after intravenous administration of Tc-99m labeled CRIP (Fig. 2); scrambled CRIP was used for comparison to demonstrate specificity of the targeting agent. A subset of animals received either captopril or captopril

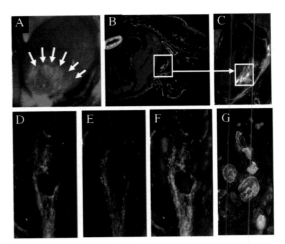

Figure 2. Imaging of proliferating myofibroblasts. *In vivo* cardiac microscopy of a two-week-old MI in a murine model shows uptake of CRIP (red) in the infarct and periinfarct zones (A, arrows). Analysis of a whole-mouse slice shows CRIP uptake in the heart (the target) and in the kidney (the main route of peptide excretion) (B). Myocardial uptake was localized in the subendocardium (C). Analysis of uptake of intravenously administered CRIP (D, red) and concurrent staining of the sections by ASMA antibody (E, red) shows colocalization of uptake was shown by overlay in longitudinal (F) and cross sections (G) demonstrating CRIP binding to myofibroblasts. MI, Myocardial infarction; CRIP, Cy5.5 RGD imaging peptide; ASMA, Alfa smooth muscle actin.

combined with losartan up to four weeks after MI to evaluate the impact of neurohumoral antagonists on myofibroblasts population and collagen deposition, and hence their role in modifying myocardial remodeling. Maximum CRIP uptake was observed in the infarct area; quantitative uptake, expressed as percent injected dose per gram (%ID/g) was highest at two weeks, sixfold higher than the myocardium of unmanipulated mice. Scrambled CRIP uptake was similar to CRIP uptake in normal myocardium. The CRIP uptake resolved by 50% in the infarct zone at three months and almost entirely disappeared at one year. However, the uptake was higher at 12 weeks in the peri-infarct zone and remote areas. The uptake was histologically traced to myofibroblasts by direct staining of CRIP with anti-Cy antibody and simultaneous staining of ASMA. Immuno-ultrastructural analysis traced by immunogold labeled anti-Cy antibody, confirmed CRIP uptake in the myofibroblasts that were rich in rough endoplasmic reticulum. *In vivo* experiments revealed CRIP binding to activated $\alpha_v\beta_{3/5}$ with an affinity of 1–3nM, but did

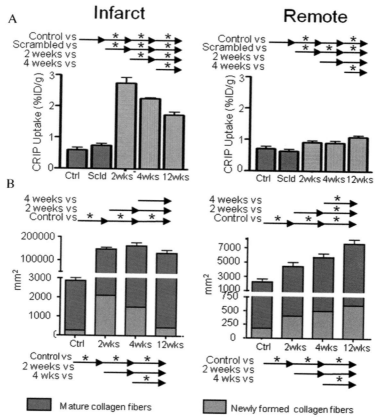

Figure 3. Characterization of radiolabeled CRIP uptake in a post-MI HF model. (A) The CRIP uptake in the infarct area was highest after two weeks and decreased over time. On the other hand, in the remote area, the uptake showed a trend towards increased uptake over time. No uptake of the technetium-scrambled CRIP was seen. (B) Polarization characterization of the collagen fibers showed that presence of the newly formed, thin collagen fibers (green) significantly correlates with CRIP uptake. *, statistically significant; CRIP, Cy5.5 RGD imaging peptide; Ctrl, control; scld, scrambled; wks, weeks.

not bind to integrins working as collagen receptors (e.g., $\alpha_I\beta_1$ or $\alpha_v\beta_1$) or platelet receptor (e.g., $\alpha_{II}\beta_3$). There was no interaction with mature collagen type I and III fibers, similar to scrambled-CRIP.

Histologic characterization of the infarcts revealed maximum myofibroblasts infiltration (expressing ASMA) at two weeks post-MI, which decreased over time (see Fig. 3). Picrosirius red polarization microscopy revealed that although the total collagen content of the infarct region remained similar over time, the thin, newly formed, yellow-green collagen fibers were reduced and correlated directly with the radiotracer uptake. Compared to the infarct zone, collagen deposition was substantially less in the remote myocardium, but overall collagen content and yellow-green thin collagen fibers increased substantially in the remote region with passage of

time; there was again a direct correlation between tracer uptake and the thin collagen fiber deposition in the remote myocardium. In addition, there was a directly proportional relationship between radiotracer uptake and ASMA-positive myofibroblasts. Correlation between radiotracer uptake and ASMA as well as thin collagen fiber areas suggests that the neocollagen production is decreased in the infarct zone and increased in remote zone over time.

A subsequent study demonstrated that treatment with one neurohumoral antagonist, such as captopril, losartan, or spironolactone, reduced the CRIP uptake by 26% in the infarct zone. All neurohumoral agents used individually were equally effective. The combination therapy reduced the uptake by 43% when any of the two agents were combined and 49%

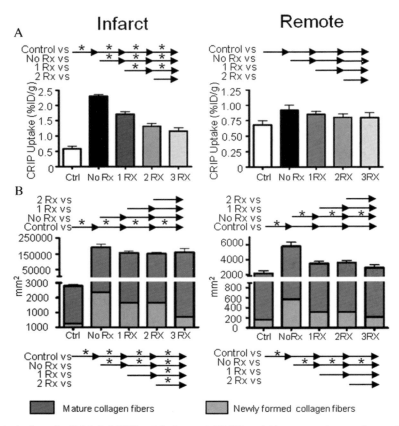

Figure 4. Characterization of radiolabeled CRIP uptake in a post-MI HF model in response to neurohumoral antagonists. CRIP uptake reduced after treatment with one, two, or three neurohumoral antagonists, including captopril, losartan, and spironolactone (A). Treatment reduced new development of collagen in remote zone and also demonstrates increased maturation of collagen in the infarct zone (B). *, statistically significant; CRIP, Cy5.5 RGD imaging peptide; MI, myocardial infarction; HF, heart failure; ctrl, control; Rx, treatment.

when all three agents were administered, demonstrating the efficacy of clinically employed therapy of HF.[29] CRIP uptake was again confirmed to be directly proportional to the number of ASMA-positive myofibroblasts and the extent of newly formed yellow-green collagen fibers. The pharmacological intervention did not decrease the deposition of total collagen content in the infarct region but newly formed collagen was substantially lowered. This was due to less production (simultaneous decrease in number of myofibroblasts) of new collagen as well as accelerated maturation of the newly formed collagen fibers. This phenomenon is represented in Figure 4 by a decrease in %ID/g CRIP uptake with pharmacologic intervention, qualitatively the same amount of total collagen, increased proportion of red-orange

fibers, and decreased presence of yellow-green immature fibers. On the other hand, there was a 30% reduction in collagen deposition in the remote myocardium by combination therapy.

To evaluate the feasibility and safety of clinical imaging of myofibroblast-associated integrin expression a nonfluorophore labeled RGD imaging peptide (RIP) was used in a small number of patients after their first episode of MI (Fig. 5).[30] RIP-based early integrin imaging was compared to the extent of fibrotic scar formation verified by late gadolinium enhanced cardiovascular magnetic resonance (CMR) imaging one year after MI. This preliminary imaging study was performed in 10 patients (ages 39–72 years, 6 male) at three and eight weeks after MI. Tc-99m labeled-RIP was injected

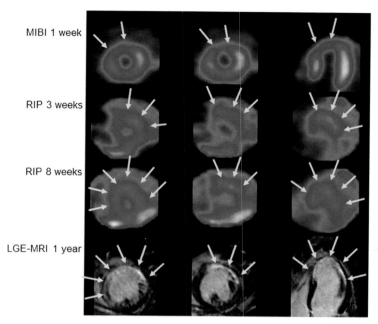

Figure 5. Clinical feasibility of RGD-based imaging in a 55-year-old male with a large mid LAD infarction. The left column shows mid-ventricular short-axis images, the middle column shows apical short axis images, the right column shows long axis images. First row: MIBI perfusion imaging at one week shows large perfusion defects in the antero-apical wall (arrows). The RIP uptake at three weeks (second row) and eight weeks (third row) extends beyond myocardial perfusion defect (arrows). RIP uptake at eight weeks is more globally spread and more intense (arrows). RIP uptake correlates with the extent of LGE-CMR-verified infarct scar at one year later (arrows). RIP imaging may allow predicting the extent of development of myocardial fibrosis. RGD, Arginine–Glycine–Aspartic Acid; LAD, Left anterior descending coronary artery; MIBI, ^{99m}Tc-Sestamibi; LGE-CMR, Late gadolinium-enhanced cardiovascular magnetic resonance imaging.

intravenously and SPECT images were acquired two hours later. Myocardial perfusion imaging was performed within one week after MI for delineation of infarct size prior to discharge. One year later all patients underwent CMR for the assessment of scar size. Image fusion and analysis software allowed comparison of both early RIP uptake and subsequent scar formation, and comparison of myocardial perfusion and RIP uptake. The RIP uptake was observed in 7 of the 10 patients at both three and eight weeks. Although the RIP uptake corresponded to areas of perfusion defects, it almost always extended beyond the infarct zone. Two of these 7 patients showed tracer uptake throughout the myocardium suggestive of global interstitial alterations. In all positive cases, RIP uptake colocalized with the extent of the scar demonstrated by MR imaging one year later. Even though more research is needed, this study provided a proof of concept for myofibroblast imaging.

Myofibroblasts and collagen deposition after MI: the good, the bad, and the ugly

Myofibroblasts in the infarct region replace the lost cardiomyocytes, which are not able to regenerate, and help produce a strong scar tissue. They also possess contractile properties and are associated with a smaller scar area, which helps to prevent infarct expansion and ventricular dilatation. On the other hand, the inexorable production of collagen from the myofibroblasts in the remote area contributes to adverse ventricular remodeling and unfavorable outcomes. Unlike in skin and other organs, myofibroblasts persist for a long time in the heart with net balance in favor of remodeling. It is of paramount importance that we understand the process of myofibroblast proliferation better and modulate the process to subdue the disadvantages without compromising the advantages. Putting the results of two studies together,[28,29] it is apparent that most of the collagen matures of a period of 12 weeks in the infarct region. Although the use of neurohumoral antagonists does not significantly decrease the amount of collagen deposition, it allows early maturation of collagen into red-orange fibers (Fig. 4). Use of all three agents resulted in maturation within four weeks post-MI, similar to what was observed at 12 weeks in untreated animals.

This may highlight the role of neurohumoral therapy in preventing infarct expansion and development of HF. Large clinical studies have demonstrated that earlier introduction of ace inhibitors (ACE-I) is more likely to prevent adverse cardiac events after MI;[31] this finding corroborates with the maximum proliferation of myofibroblasts (or CRIP uptake) within the first two weeks of acute events. In contrast to the infarct zone, the extent of myofibroblastic proliferation in the remote region is much smaller and neurohumoral agents are able to substantially contain the release of new collagen fibers and eventually restrict the total amount of collagen deposition, effectively preventing evolution of cardiac adverse remodeling. These studies of myofibroblast imaging presented here have contributed to understanding of the mechanisms of myocardial alterations in HF.

Conclusions

Molecular imaging is the only strategy that allows targeting and elucidation of subcellular processes in a living organism. The better knowledge of a pathogenetic process allows novel avenues for the development of targeted imaging. The feasibility of targeting subcellular events allows enhanced understanding of pathogenesis. It is proposed that molecular imaging in research should be increasingly utilized not only for diagnostic purposes, but also for uncovering the intricacies of the processes involved in disease development.[32]

Acknowledgments

Dedicated to the memory of the late Lovhaug Dagfinn PhD, who helped develop the CRIP and RIP imaging agents described herein for myofibroblast imaging. Hans de Haas was partially supported by grants from the Dutch Heart Foundation (Dr. E. Dekker Scholarship) and the foundation "De Drie Lichten." The authors gratefully acknowledge all colleague scientists for their contributions in this research area.

Conflicts of interest

The authors declare no conflicts of interest.

References

1. Bujak, M. & N.G. Frangogiannis. 2007. The role of TGF-beta signaling in myocardial infarction and cardiac remodeling. *Cardiovasc. Res.* **74:** 184–195.
2. Blankesteijn, W.M., E. Creemers, E. Lutgens, *et al.* 2001. Dynamics of cardiac wound healing following myocardial infarction: observations in genetically altered mice. *Acta Physiol. Scand.* **173:** 75–82.
3. Desmoulière, A., A. Geinoz, F. Gabbiani, *et al.* 1993. Transforming growth factor-beta 1 induces alpha-smooth muscle actin expression in granulation tissue myofibroblasts and in quiescent and growing cultured fibroblasts. *J. Cell. Biol.* **122:** 103–111.
4. Miettinen, P.J., R. Ebner, A.R. Lopez, *et al.* 1994. TGF-beta induced transdifferentiation of mammary epithelial cells to mesenchymal cells: involvement of type I receptors. *J. Cell. Biol.* **127:** 2021–2036.
5. Sun, Y., M.F. Kiani, A.E. Postlethwaite, *et al.* 2002. Infarct scar as living tissue. *Basic Res. Cardiol.* **97:** 343–347.
6. Cleutjens, J.P., W.M. Blankesteijn, M.J. Daemen, *et al.* 1999. The infarcted myocardium: simply dead tissue, or a lively target for therapeutic interventions. *Cardiovasc. Res.* **44:** 232–241.
7. Smith-Mungo, L.I. & H.M. Kagan. 1998. Lysyl oxidase: properties, regulation and multiple functions in biology. *Matrix. Biol.* **16:** 387–398.
8. Sun, Y. 2000. Infarct scar: a dynamic tissue. *Cardiovasc. Res.* **46:** 250–256.
9. van den Borne, S.W.M., J. Diez, W.M. Blankesteijn, *et al.* 2010. Myocardial remodeling after infarction: the role of myofibroblasts. *Nat. Rev. Cardiol.* **7:** 30–37.
10. Rosenkranz, S., M. Flesch, K. Amann, *et al.* 2002. Alterations of beta-adrenergic signaling and cardiac hypertrophy in transgenic mice overexpressing TGF-beta(1). *Am. J. Physiol. Heart. Circ. Physiol.* **283:** H1253–H1262.
11. Eyden, B. 2005. The myofibroblast: a study of normal, reactive and neoplastic tissues, with an emphasis on ultrastructure. Part 1-normal and reactive cells. *J. Submicrosc. Cytol. Pathol.* **37:** 109–204.
12. Hinz, B., S.H. Phan, V.J. Thannickal, *et al.* 2007. The myofibroblast: one function, multiple origins. *Am. J. Path.* **170:** 1807–1816.
13. Blankesteijn, W.M., Y.P. Essers-Janssen, M.J. Verluyten, *et al.* 1997. A homologue of Drosophila tissue polarity gene frizzled is expressed in migrating myofibroblasts in the infarcted rat heart. *Nat. Med.* **3:** 541–544.
14. Wynn, T.A. 2008. Cellular and molecular mechanisms of fibrosis. *J. Pathol.* **214:** 199–210.
15. Hinz, B. 2006. Masters and servants of the force: the role of matrix adhesions in myofibroblast force perception and transmission. *Eur. J. Cell Biol.* **85:** 175–181.
16. Hong, H.H., M.I. Uzel, C. Duan, *et al.* 1999. Regulation of lysyl oxidase, collagen, and connective tissue growth factor by TGF-beta1 and detection in human gingiva. *Lab. Invest.* **79:** 1655–1667.

17. Weber, K.T. 1997. Extracellular matrix remodeling in heart failure: a role for de novo angiotensin II generation. *Circulation* **96:** 4065–4082.
18. Harada, K., T. Sugaya, K. Murakami, *et al.* 1999. Angiotensin II type 1A receptor knockout mice display less left ventricular remodeling and improved survival after myocardial infarction. *Circulation* **100:** 2093–2099.
19. Pfeffer, M.A., K. Swedberg, C.B. Granger, *et al.* 2003. Effects of candesartan on mortality and morbidity in patients with chronic heart failure: the CHARM-Overall programme. *Lancet.* **362:** 759–766.
20. Pitt, B., P.A. Poole-Wilson, R. Segal, *et al.* 2000. Effect of losartan compared with captopril on mortality in patients with symptomatic heart failure: randomised trial–the Losartan Heart Failure Survival Study ELITE II. *Lancet.* **355:** 1582–1587.
21. Cohn, J.N. & G. Tognoni. 2001. A randomized trial of the angiotensin-receptor blocker valsartan in chronic heart failure. *N. Engl. J. Med.* **345:** 1667–1675.
22. The CONSENSUS Trial Study Group. 1987. Effects of enalapril on mortality in severe congestive heart failure. Results of the Cooperative North Scandinavian Enalapril Survival Study (CONSENSUS). *N. Engl. J. Med.* **316:** 1429–1435.
23. The SOLVD Investigators. 1991. Effect of enalapril on survival in patients with reduced left ventricular ejection fractions and congestive heart failure. *N. Engl. J. Med.* **325:** 293–302.
24. Verjans, J.W.H., D. Lovhaug, N. Narula, *et al.* 2008. Noninvasive imaging of angiotensin receptors after myocardial infarction. *JACC Cardiovasc. Imaging* **1:** 354–362.
25. Dilsizian, V., W.C. Eckelman, M.L. Loredo, *et al.* 2007. Evidence for tissue angiotensin-converting enzyme in explanted hearts of ischemic cardiomyopathy using targeted radiotracer technique. *J. Nucl. Med.* **48:** 182–187.
26. Dilsizian, V., T.K. Zynda, A. Petrov, *et al.* 2012. Molecular imaging of human angiotensin converting enzyme-1 expression in transgenic rats with hybrid micro SPECT/CT. *JACC. Cardiovasc. Imaging.* In Press.
27. Asano, Y., H. Ihn, K. Yamane, *et al.* 2005. Increased expression of integrin alpha(v)beta3 contributes to the establishment of autocrine TGF-beta signaling in scleroderma fibroblasts. *J. Immunol.* **175:** 7708–7718.
28. van den Borne, S.W.M., S. Isobe, J.W. Verjans, *et al.* 2008. Molecular imaging of interstitial alterations in remodeling myocardium after myocardial infarction. *J. Am. Coll. Cardiol.* **52:** 2017–2028.
29. van den Borne, S.W.M., S. Isobe, H.R. Zandbergen, *et al.* 2009. Molecular imaging for efficacy of pharmacologic intervention in myocardial remodeling. *JACC. Cardiovasc. Imaging* **2:** 187–198.
30. Verjans, J., S. Wolters, W. Laufer, *et al.* 2010. Early molecular imaging of interstitial changes in patients after myocardial infarction: comparison with delayed contrast-enhanced magnetic resonance imaging. *J. Nucl. Cardiol.* **17:** 1065–1072.
31. Gruppo Italiano per lo Studio della Sopravvivenza nell'infarto Miocardico. 1994. GISSI-3: effects of lisinopril and transdermal glyceryl trinitrate singly and together on 6-week mortality and ventricular function after acute myocardial infarction. *Lancet* **343:** 1115–1122.
32. Narula, J. & V. Dilsizian. 2008. From better understood pathogenesis to superior molecular imaging, and back. *JACC. Cardiovasc. Imaging* **1:** 406–409.

Ann. N.Y. Acad. Sci. ISSN 0077-8923

ANNALS OF THE NEW YORK ACADEMY OF SCIENCES

Issue: *Evolving Challenges in Promoting Cardiovascular Health*

Molecular targets in heart failure gene therapy: current controversies and translational perspectives

Victor Kairouz,[1] Larissa Lipskaia,[2] Roger J. Hajjar,[2] and Elie R. Chemaly[2]

[1]Department of Internal Medicine, University at Buffalo School of Medicine and Biomedical Sciences, Erie County Medical Center, Buffalo, New York. [2]Cardiovascular Research Center, Mount Sinai School of Medicine, New York, New York

Address for correspondence: Roger J. Hajjar, M.D., Cardiovascular Research Center, Mount Sinai School of Medicine, One Gustave L. Levy Place Box 1030, New York, NY 10029. roger.hajjar@mssm.edu

Use of gene therapy for heart failure is gaining momentum as a result of the recent successful completion of phase II of the Calcium Upregulation by Percutaneous Administration of Gene Therapy in Cardiac Disease (CUPID) trial, which showed clinical safety and efficacy of an adeno-associated viral vector expressing sarco-endoplasmic reticulum calcium ATPase (SERCA2a). Resorting to gene therapy allows the manipulation of molecular targets not presently amenable to pharmacologic modulation. This short review focuses on the molecular targets of heart failure gene therapy that have demonstrated translational potential. At present, most of these targets are related to calcium handling in the cardiomyocyte. They include SERCA2a, phospholamban, S100A1, ryanodine receptor, and the inhibitor of the protein phosphatase 1. Other targets related to cAMP signaling are reviewed, such as adenylyl cyclase. MicroRNAs are emerging as novel therapeutic targets and convenient vectors for gene therapy, particularly in heart disease. We propose a discussion of recent advances and controversies in key molecular targets of heart failure gene therapy.

Keywords: heart failure; gene therapy; calcium handling; phospholamban; adenylyl cyclase; protein phosphatase 1

Introduction

The emergence of gene therapy as a promising strategy to treat heart failure is a multifactorial phenomenon. First, there is an unmet need to develop effective treatments aimed at decreasing the morbidity and mortality of heart failure, a highly prevalent problem associated with a grim prognosis despite continuing therapeutic progress.[1,2] Second, attractive therapeutic targets were identified and validated, such as the sarco-endoplasmic reticulum calcium ATPase (SERCA2a),[1] without available and effective pharmacologic modulators. The search for pharmacologic agents to modulate these targets was undertaken in parallel with the development of gene therapy tools. Isatroxime is a promising stimulator of SERCA2a recently evaluated in a clinical trial; of note, isatroxime is also an inhibitor of the sodium–potassium ATPase.[3,4]

However, the recent successful completion of a phase II clinical trial of gene therapy to enhance the myocardial expression of SERCA2a in patients with heart failure[5] propels gene therapy forward in the clinical armamentarium as a safe and effective approach.

The subject of gene therapy in heart failure has been extensively reviewed.[1,6,7] The purpose of this brief review is to provide a focused update on the current translational advances and controversies related to the molecular targets in the gene therapy of heart failure.

Multiple molecular mechanisms were targeted by gene therapy in animal models of heart failure.[1,6,7] The common aim of these studies was to restore the function of cardiomyocytic signaling pathways consistently shown to be defective in heart failure, such as β-adrenergic signaling and calcium handling. Other studies targeted distinct processes, such as cell survival pathways.[7] A common strategy of these studies was to use recombinant DNA-based vectors to modulate gene expression.

doi: 10.1111/j.1749-6632.2012.06520.x

In this setting, it is important to note that vector-based modulation of molecular pathways is also a strategy for proof-of-concept studies in cardiovascular physiology and pathophysiology. Progression from vector-based gene expression modulation to clinical gene therapy is dependent both on the therapeutic potential of the target gene and on the lack of safe and effective pharmacological approaches—for example, proteine kinase C was modulated by viral vectors and pharmacologic agents in recent studies.[8,9] Thus, our review will focus on therapeutic targets pertaining to gene therapy with translational potential.

Viral vectors

Viral vectors (reviewed by Kawase *et al.*[7]) have been effective at infecting various cell types, including cardiac myocytes. Recombinant adenoviral vectors were used early on to infect the heart, with reasonable transgene expression, although the duration of expression was limited to weeks due to immune response generated against the remaining viral genes. Lentiviruses, which can infect postmitotic cells, have also been used. However, their integration within the genome is a concern because they can integrate within or near a tumor suppressing or promoting area and cause unchecked growth and division. Adeno-associated viruses (AAVs) have emerged as ideal vectors for infecting the myocardium in the setting of heart failure. Their characteristics include long-term transgene expression and minimal immune response. In addition, recombinant AAVs used for gene therapy do not integrate in the host genome (as compared to wild-type AAV). Their small size is, in addition, an advantage when the need arises for infusing them through the coronary arteries. One drawback of AAVs, however, is their inability to incorporate more than 4.7 kb of genetic material. Because of their transduction ability and safety profile, AAV vectors have gained a strong foothold not only in the treatment of cardiovascular diseases but also of other organ diseases.

Therapeutic targets related to calcium handling in the cardiomyocyte

The abnormal calcium handling in the failing cardiomyocyte is complex. It involves mainly sarcoplasmic reticumlum (SR) Ca^{2+} leak through the ryanodine receptor (RyR) and decreased SR Ca^{2+} uptake associated with a decline of SERCA2a expression and activity—together, these result in reduced SR Ca^{2+} loading.[6] This is a critical component of the impaired mechanical performance of failing hearts,[6] in addition to arrhythmogenesis.[10] Calcium-handling proteins and their regulators are thus promising therapeutic targets in heart failure.[6]

SERCA2a overexpression

The overexpression of SERCA2a by gene therapy in heart failure is a historical model, beginning with the finding of defective calcium handling associated with reduced SERCA2a expression in failing cardiac myocytes and progressing to a clinical trial where an AAV overexpressing SERCA2a was administered to heart failure patients.[5,7]

The multiple steps of this process, involving target validation, the development of gene therapy vectors and delivery methods, along with the testing of animal models of heart failure, have been reviewed elsewhere.[11] Along with the demonstration of improved myocardial mechanical function, the overexpression of SERCA2a had multiple effects, including improved myocardial energetics, endothelial function, and coronary flow.[7] The antiarrhythmic effects of SERCA2a overexpression were demonstrated in acute ischemia-reperfusion.[10] In chronic heart failure after myocardial infarction in rats, overexpression of SERCA2a was associated with a reduction of spontaneous and provoked ventricular arrhythmia, along with a reduction in calcium leak from the SR.[12] The latter findings confirm the clinical safety of SERCA2a gene therapy in the arrhythmia-prone heart failure population.[12]

Phase II of the Calcium Upregulation by Percutaneous Administration of Gene Therapy in Cardiac Disease (CUPID) study was recently published.[5] This trial confirmed the clinical safety of SERCA2a overexpression by gene therapy previously demonstrated in phase I.[13] Therapeutic efficacy was demonstrated in several clinical, biological, and echocardiographic indicators of heart failure.[5] In particular, patients receiving the highest dose of AAV1–SERCA2a demonstrated improvement in the six-minute walk test and in left ventricular end-systolic volume, along with reduced hospitalization stay and incidence of prespecified multiple cardiovascular events.[5]

Other ongoing clinical trials of overexpression of SERCA2a in heart failure were reviewed recently.[7] They include (1) a trial in which AAV1–SERCA2a gene transfer will be performed one month after placement of a left ventricular assist device (LVAD), with the endpoint being the ability to wean the LVAD; and (2) a trial where AAV1–SERCA2a gene transfer will be performed in patients with Class III/IV heart failure, and cardiac structural parameters will be examined six months after gene transfer.

Enhancing activity of SERCA2a through modulation of phospholamban

The therapeutic implications of the interaction between SERCA2s and phospholamban (PLB) in heart failure were first derived from studies on transgenic mice lacking PLB in which the progression of heart failure was abrogated.[14] Multiple gene therapy studies were conducted *in vitro* and *in vivo* using viral vectors with antisense RNA or shRNA to downregulate PLB.[15,16] Other studies used dominant-negative forms of PLB, designed to keep PLB in the inactive pentameric form.[17] Since phosphorylation of PLB on serin-16 prevents the inhibition on SERCA2a, a pseudophosphorylated form of PLB (the S16E mutant), overexpressed by gene therapy, demonstrated improved left ventricular function in animal models of heart failure, including a large animal model.[18]

However, several challenges related to the modulation of PLB as a therapeutic target have emerged from recent studies.

First, it is known that PLB only modulates the calcium-dependence of SERCA2a activity, that is, the affinity of the enzyme for calcium (K_{Ca}); therefore, PLB has no impact on maximal SERCA2a activity that occurs at saturating calcium concentrations.[19]

Second, in one report, PLB knockout mice progressed to heart failure after aortic constriction, similarly to control animals.[20] Although PLB ablation seems promising in rodents, complete ablation of PLB may not be beneficial in humans. Humans with PLB null-mutations suffer from lethal dilated cardiomyopathy.[21] We must accompany our citation of this work[21] by a word of caution: the L39Stop mutation of PLB does not equate with PLB ablation, and may in fact be a form of PLB that exerts untoward effects.[22] Moreover, the cardiac cellular toxicity of a therapy involving short hairpin RNA against PLB in dogs was recently reported, which was attributed to an adverse interference of shRNA with microRNA pathways.[22]

Third, the S16E mutant of PLB lacks the possibility of further phosphorylation at the serine 16 residue,[19] which may limit its therapeutic applicability. Recently, a systematic approach was undertaken to identify mutants of PLB that possess an affinity to SERCA comparable to the wild-type PLB, while having less inhibitory potential and retaining the possibility of being phosphorylated.[23] It has been shown that PLB phosphorylation does not lead to a dissociation of the SERCA–PLB complex; instead, PLB remains bound to SERCA, but its inhibitory effect on SERCA is reduced by phosphorylation.[19] This opens the possibility of using PLB mutants as a therapy by having a less inhibitory mutant act as a partial antagonist to wild-type PLB, thus displacing wild-type PLB from SERCA.[19] The physiologic ratio of PLB/SERCA is 5/1, and a recent study showed a potential for increased SERCA activity with PLB mutants present in molar concentrations at least as abundant as wild-type PLB.[19] Studies are underway to determine whether these *in vitro* ratios can be achieved *in vivo* in animal models of heart failure.

Finally, while overexpression of PLB mutants may be beneficial, this may lead to an increase in the total amount of PLB in the cardiomyocyte. Existing literature demonstrates a reduction in cardiomyocyte function associated with the overexpression of PLB, whether transgenic approach or by adenoviral vector.[21,24] Increase in PLB expression was found in diabetic cardiomyopathy and in the setting of resistin overexpression.[25]

Considering that PLB is only a 52 amino acids peptide, one can expect, at least theoretically, to target pharmacologically the SERCA2a–PLB interaction.

Protein phosphatase 1, its endogenous inhibitor and regulator I1, and the activated form of I1, I1c

The protein phosphatase 1 (PP1)–I1 couple represents a central and complex mechanism of regulation of phosphorylation and dephosphorylation in the cardiac myocyte and in other cell types, and was recently and extensively reviewed by Wittkopper *et al.*[26] This molecular couple has emerged as an attractive therapeutic target for heart failure, due to the increased levels and activity of PP1, together with reduced levels and activity of I1, in heart failure.[26] PP1 dephosphorylates PLB at the serine 16 residue (Fig. 1); thus,

23. Ha, K.N., N.J. Traaseth, R. Verardi, *et al.* 2007. Controlling the inhibition of the sarcoplasmic Ca2+-ATPase by tuning phospholamban structural dynamics. *J. Biol. Chem.* **282:** 37205–37214.

24. Kadambi, V.J., S. Ponniah, J.M. Harrer, *et al.* 1996. Cardiac-specific overexpression of phospholamban alters calcium kinetics and resultant cardiomyocyte mechanics in transgenic mice. *J. Clin. Invest.* **97:** 533–539.

25. Chemaly, E.R., L. Hadri, S. Zhang, *et al.* 2011. Long-term in vivo resistin overexpression induces myocardial dysfunction and remodeling in rats. *J. Mol. Cell Cardiol.* **51:** 144–155.

26. Wittkopper, K., D. Dobrev, T. Eschenhagen & A. El-Armouche. 2011. Phosphatase-1 inhibitor-1 in physiological and pathological beta-adrenoceptor signalling. *Cardiovasc. Res.* **91:** 392–401.

27. Pathak, A., F. del Monte, W. Zhao, *et al.* 2005. Enhancement of cardiac function and suppression of heart failure progression by inhibition of protein phosphatase 1. *Circ. Res.* **96:** 756–766.

28. Kho, C., A. Lee, D. Jeong, *et al.* 2011. SUMO1-dependent modulation of SERCA2a in heart failure. *Nature* **477:** 601–605.

29. Pleger, S.T., C. Shan, J. Ksienzyk, *et al.* 2011. Cardiac AAV9-S100A1 gene therapy rescues post-ischemic heart failure in a preclinical large animal model. *Sci. Transl. Med.* **3:** 92ra64.

30. Belmonte, S.L., K.B. Margulies & B.C. Blaxall. 2011. S100A1: another step toward therapeutic development for heart failure. *J. Am. Coll. Cardiol.* **58:** 974–976.

31. Brinks, H., D. Rohde, M. Voelkers, *et al.* 2011. S100A1 genetically targeted therapy reverses dysfunction of human failing cardiomyocytes. *J. Am. Coll. Cardiol.* **58:** 966–973.

32. Feldman, D.S., C.A. Carnes, W.T. Abraham & M.R. Bristow. 2005. Mechanisms of disease: beta-adrenergic receptors–alterations in signal transduction and pharmacogenomics in heart failure. *Nat. Clin. Pract. Cardiovasc. Med.* **2:** 475–483.

33. Lipskaia, L., H. Ly, Y. Kawase, *et al.* 2007. Treatment of heart failure by calcium cycling gene therapy. *Future Cardiol.* **3:** 413–423.

34. Vinge, L.E., P.W. Raake & W.J. Koch. 2008. Gene therapy in heart failure. *Circ. Res.* **102:** 1458–1470.

35. Gao, M.H., N.C. Lai, D.M. Roth, *et al.* 1999. Adenylylcyclase increases responsiveness to catecholamine stimulation in transgenic mice. *Circulation* **99:** 1618–1622.

36. Regitz-Zagrosek, V., R. Hertrampf, C. Steffen, *et al.* 1994. Myocardial cyclic AMP and norepinephrine content in human heart failure. *Eur. Heart J.* **15**(Suppl. D): 7–13.

37. Lohse, M.J., S. Engelhardt & T. Eschenhagen. 2003. What is the role of beta-adrenergic signaling in heart failure? *Circ. Res.* **93:** 896–906.

38. Ostrom, R.S., S.R. Post & P.A. Insel. 2000. Stoichiometry and compartmentation in G protein-coupled receptor signaling: implications for therapeutic interventions involving G(s). *J. Pharmacol. Exp. Ther.* **294:** 407–412.

39. Defer, N., M. Best-Belpomme & J. Hanoune. 2000. Tissue specificity and physiological relevance of various isoforms of adenylyl cyclase. *Am J. Physiol. Renal Physiol.* **279:** F400–416.

40. Hanoune, J. & N. Defer. 2001. Regulation and role of adenylyl cyclase isoforms. *Annu. Rev. Pharmacol. Toxicol.* **41:** 145–174.

41. Puceat, M., C. Bony, M. Jaconi & G. Vassort. 1998. Specific activation of adenylyl cyclase V by a purinergic agonist. *FEBS Letters* **431:** 189–194.

42. Stark, J.C., S.F. Haydock, R. Foo, *et al.* 2004. Effect of overexpressed adenylyl cyclase VI on beta 1- and beta 2-adrenoceptor responses in adult rat ventricular myocytes. *Br. J. Pharmacol.* **143:** 465–476.

43. Hu, C.L., R. Chandra, H. Ge, *et al.* 2009. Adenylyl cyclase type 5 protein expression during cardiac development and stress. *Am. J. Physiol. Heart Circ. Physiol.* **297:** H1776–H1782.

44. Espinasse, I., V. Iourgenko, C. Richer, *et al.* 1999. Decreased type VI adenylyl cyclase mRNA concentration and Mg(2+)-dependent adenylyl cyclase activities and unchanged type V adenylyl cyclase mRNA concentration and Mn(2+)-dependent adenylyl cyclase activities in the left ventricle of rats with myocardial infarction and longstanding heart failure. *Cardiovasc. Res.* **42:** 87–98.

45. Tepe, N.M., J.N. Lorenz, A. Yatani, *et al.* 1999. Altering the receptor-effector ratio by transgenic overexpression of type V adenylyl cyclase: enhanced basal catalytic activity and function without increased cardiomyocyte beta-adrenergic signalling. *Biochemistry* **38:** 16706–16713.

46. Vatner, S.F., L. Yan, Y. Ishikawa, *et al.* 2009. Adenylyl cyclase type 5 disruption prolongs longevity and protects the heart against stress. *Circ. J.* **73:** 195–200.

47. Okumura, S., G. Takagi, J. Kawabe, *et al.* 2003. Disruption of type 5 adenylyl cyclase gene preserves cardiac function against pressure overload. *Proc. Natl. Acad. Sci. U. S. A.* **100:** 9986–9990.

48. Tang, T., H.K. Hammond, A. Firth, *et al.* 2011. Adenylyl cyclase 6 improves calcium uptake and left ventricular function in aged hearts. *J. Am. Coll. Cardiol.* **57:** 1846–1855.

49. Gao, M.H., T. Tang, T. Guo, *et al.* 2008. Adenylyl cyclase type VI increases Akt activity and phospholamban phosphorylation in cardiac myocytes. *J. Biol. Chem.* **283:** 33527–33535.

50. Gao, M.H., T. Tang, A. Miyanohara, *et al.* 2010. beta(1)-Adrenergic receptor vs adenylyl cyclase 6 expression in cardiac myocytes: differences in transgene localization and intracellular signaling. *Cell. Signal.* **22:** 584–589.

51. Lipskaia, L., N. Defer, G. Esposito, *et al.* 2000. Enhanced cardiac function in transgenic mice expressing a Ca(2+)-stimulated adenylyl cyclase. *Circ. Res.* **86:** 795–801.

52. Lipskaia, L., N. Mougenot, A. Jacquet, *et al.* 2011. Compartmentalization of cAMP increase at the level of sarcoplasmic reticulum results in dilated and hypertrophic cardiomyopathy in aged transgenic mice. *Eur. Heart J.* **32**(Suppl. 1): 999.

53. Georget, M., P. Mateo, G. Vandecasteele, *et al.* 2002. Augmentation of cardiac contractility with no change in L-type Ca2+ current in transgenic mice with a cardiac-directed expression of the human adenylyl cyclase type 8 (AC8). *FASEB J.* **16:** 1636–1638.

54. Georget, M., P. Mateo, G. Vandecasteele, *et al.* 2003. Cyclic AMP compartmentation due to increased cAMP-phosphodiesterase activity in transgenic mice with a cardiac-directed expression of the human adenylyl cyclase type 8 (AC8). *FASEB J.* **17:** 1380–1391.

55. Levin, S.D., D.W. Taft, C.S. Brandt, *et al.* 2011. Vstm3 is a member of the CD28 family and an important modulator of T-cell function. *Eur. J. Immunol.* **41:** 902–915.

56. Lyon, A.R., M. Sato, R.J. Hajjar, *et al.* 2008. Gene therapy: targeting the myocardium. *Heart (British Cardiac Society)* **94:** 89–99.

57. Ghadge, S.K., S. Muhlstedt, C. Ozcelik & M. Bader. 2011. SDF-1alpha as a therapeutic stem cell homing factor in myocardial infarction. *Pharmacol. Ther.* **129:** 97–108.

58. Pyo, R.T., J. Sui, A. Dhume, *et al.* 2006. CXCR4 modulates contractility in adult cardiac myocytes. *J. Mol. Cell Cardiol.* **41:** 834–844.

59. Chen, J., E. Chemaly, L. Liang, *et al.* 2010. Effects of CXCR4 gene transfer on cardiac function after ischemia-reperfusion injury. *Am. J. Pathol.* **176:** 1705–1715.

60. LaRocca, T.J., M. Schwarzkopf, P. Altman, *et al.* 2010. beta2-Adrenergic receptor signaling in the cardiac myocyte is modulated by interactions with CXCR4. *J. Cardiovasc. Pharmacol.* **56:** 548–559.

61. van Rooij, E. 2011. The art of microRNA research. *Circ. Res.* **108:** 219–234.

62. Karakikes, I., A. Chaanine, J. Kim, *et al.* 2010. Abstract 20916: therapeutic cardiac-targeted delivery of Mir-1 reverses hypertrophy and preserves cardiac function in a pressure overload animal model. *Circulation* **122:** A20916.

Ann. N.Y. Acad. Sci. ISSN 0077-8923

ANNALS OF THE NEW YORK ACADEMY OF SCIENCES
Issue: *Evolving Challenges in Promoting Cardiovascular Health*

Engineered arterial models to correlate blood flow to tissue biological response

Jordi Martorell,[1,2] Pablo Santomá,[1,2] José J. Molins,[1] Andrés A. García-Granada,[3] José A. Bea,[4] Elazer R. Edelman,[2,5] and Mercedes Balcells[2,6]

[1]Department of Chemical Engineering, IQS, Universitat Ramon Llull, Barcelona, Spain. [2]Harvard-MIT Biomedical Engineering Center, Massachusetts Institute of Technology, Cambridge, Massachusetts. [3]Department of Industrial Engineering, IQS, Universitat Ramon Llull, Barcelona, Spain. [4]Department of Mechanical Engineering, Universidad de Zaragoza, Spain. [5]Cardiology Division, Brigham and Women's Hospital, Boston, Massachusetts. [6]Bioengineering Department, IQS, Universitat Ramon Llull, Barcelona, Spain

Address for correspondence: Mercedes Balcells, Harvard-MIT Division of Health Sciences and Technology, 77 Massachusetts Avenue, Building E25-438, Cambridge, MA 02139. merche@mit.edu

This paper reviews how biomedical engineers, in collaboration with physicians, biologists, chemists, physicists, and mathematicians, have developed models to explain how the impact of vascular interventions on blood flow predicts subsequent vascular repair. These models have become increasingly sophisticated and precise, propelling us toward optimization of cardiovascular therapeutics in general and personalizing treatments for patients with cardiovascular disease.

Keywords: atherosclerosis; endothelium; blood flow

Atherosclerosis, the most common cause of disease and death in the developed world, affects all arterial beds. The clinical treatment for atherosclerosis has evolved tremendously over many decades, with percutaneous interventions such as stents and/or grafts becoming almost a commodity in patient care. Despite technological improvements, restenosis, and stent and graft thrombosis continue to hamper the success of the implants. It has been suggested that only modifications of interventions personalized to individual state and vascular geometries can prevent flow- and drug-related postimplantation complications. Several *in vitro* and *ex vivo* models have been developed to explain partially the molecular mechanisms of atherogenesis, thrombosis, or restenosis. It is now possible to tailor these models to include patient-specific characteristics in the search for personalized solutions.

In vitro flow chambers

The endothelium is a unique organ. As a monolayer of cells exposed to blood flow, the endothelium expresses an ordered array of biochemical regulators that ensure blood fluidity along and through the vessels, nutrient transport, and an appropriate control of coagulation if the lining integrity is compromised. Endothelial cells are constantly in direct contact with blood flow and are flow sensitive. Hence, the expression of proteins is triggered by and depends upon local hemodynamics. As the vascular system is a closed universe, the interaction between flow and the endothelium can be studied in a specific fashion and controlled environments using *in vitro* and *ex vivo* model systems—flow chambers.

In 2002, Blackman, García-Cardeña, and Gimbrone introduced the dynamic flow system (DFS)[1] as a culmination of decades of research on the effects of flow on endothelial cell biology.[2,3] The DFS consists of tissue culture wells seeded with functional endothelial cells under controlled humidity, temperature, and CO_2 levels, and a medium feeding system. A conical device coupled to a motor rotates and generates a controlled flow over cultured endothelial cells. Endothelial cells in static conditions act differently than those subject to flow. Arterial flow reshapes the cytoskeleton and reduces eNOS

doi: 10.1111/j.1749-6632.2012.06518.x
Ann. N.Y. Acad. Sci. 1254 (2012) 51–56 © 2012 New York Academy of Sciences.

mRNA expression. Later, Dr. Gimbrone's group used the DFS to define athero-prone and athero-protective waveforms[4] and showed how endothelial cells exposed to athero-prone waveforms expressed a proinflammatory phenotype, including increase of NF-κB, VCAM and e-Selectin, among others. Our group reported similar findings in 2005 using a different flow chamber, proving that the activity of eNOS and production of prostaglandins was dependent on flow frequency.[5] Here, endothelial cells were seeded in silicone tubular structures and connected to a perfusion loop. Media circulated through the system using a programmable pump that delivered well-defined and physiologically matched velocities and shear stresses.

Ex vivo flow chambers

Much earlier, Badimon *et al.* designed the first *ex vivo* chamber,[6] using de-endothelialized swine arteries, to prove the relevance of shear rates on platelet deposition. Replacing the de-endothelialized artery by a collagen strip proved the key role of collagen in postinterventional thrombogenicity. This 1986 *ex vivo* model is still a valid tool to evaluate the effects of anticoagulant drugs[7] or other thrombogenicity relevant questions. This model, however, does not recapitulate the interaction between smooth muscle cells and the remaining endothelial cells nor the full architecture of the vessel. Another interesting approach was introduced in 2002, when Kolandaivelu and Edelman designed an *ex vivo* system to study stent thrombogenicity.[8,9] A peristaltic pump is substituted by a rotor and the inertial flow imposed is customizable so the waveforms are totally controlled. This model has been used to study and optimize stent designs and enlighten different aspects of stent thrombosis.[10]

Cellular co-culture

Endothelial cells are not only in direct contact with blood flow but interact with their underlying cellular neighbors. Many of the questions one may ask cannot be answered if considering one cell type alone. Balcells *et al.* proved that the mTOR pathway in endothelial cells is promoted by alterations in flow,[11] but to a far lesser extent when intact vascular smooth muscle cells were present in the system. These findings confirm the importance of the big picture in understanding endothelial function. At a microscopic scale, several groups have applied surface patterning and engineered test chambers to study cell–cell crosstalk. A number of strategies have been developed; Chen's bow-ties or Bhatia's micropatterned cocultures are good examples. Chen and colleagues showed how VE-cadherin is responsible for contact growth inhibition and the role of this molecule in regulating how cells adhere to the extracellular matrix.[12] Bhatia and colleagues engineered several microscale devices to study cell–cell interaction in liver cells. Liver sinusoidal endothelial cells (LSEC) have a very particular phenotype that is hard to maintain *in vitro*. To maintain phenotype, Bhatia's group co-cultured LSECs with hepatocytes and fibroblasts on collagen.[13] These findings suggest that the optimal strategy to create a physiologically relevant *in vitro* model depends on the cell type and the *in vivo* micro- and macro-environment simulated. There is no unique solution to how many variables should be included when engineering biological models.

Computational models

Computational models have gained increasing acceptance as valuable tools to predict physical, chemical, and biological phenomena in arteries. Computational fluid dynamics (CFD) simulations can predict with micrometric precision several physical and biological variables, such as velocity, shear stress, and drug distribution profiles. This is particularly important in stent design, where biological analytical methods cannot provide the required precision to define micrometer-based events. There is an increasing interest in understanding how micro-alterations and separation in flow caused by stent struts may affect local drug delivery[14,15] and stent thrombogenicity.[10] Recent studies[16] couple the computational results with *in vivo* experience, but this is only possible when classic mass transport equations and molecule-specific uptake kinetics are considered together and with accurate input parameters derived and validated from *in vivo* conditions[16,17] CFD simulations are limited by their input validity, but when validated, they offer a platform for repeatable, quantifiable assay of effects across a spectrum of dependent parameters, device and formulation modifications, and environmental conditions—a feature unachievable with biological and animal testing. Computational models have become so helpful that the U.S. Food and Drug Administration is consid-

Ann. N.Y. Acad. Sci. ISSN 0077-8923

ANNALS OF THE NEW YORK ACADEMY OF SCIENCES

Issue: *Evolving Challenges in Promoting Cardiovascular Health*

A bird's-eye view of cell therapy and tissue engineering for cardiac regeneration

Carolina Soler-Botija,[1] Juli R. Bagó,[2,3] and Antoni Bayes-Genis[1,2,4]

[1]Heart Failure and Cardiac Regeneration (ICREC) Research Program, Health Research Institute Germans Trias i Pujol (IGTP), Cardiology Service, Hospital Universitari Germans Trias i Pujol, Badalona, Spain. [2]Networking Biomedical Research Center on Bioengineering, Biomaterials and Nanomedicine (CIBER-BBN), Barcelona, Spain. [3]Cardiovascular Research Center (CSIC-ICCC), Barcelona, Spain. [4]Department of Medicine, Autonomous University Barcelona, Barcelona, Spain

Address for correspondence: Antoni Bayes-Genis, M.D., Ph.D., F.E.S.C., I.C.R.E.C. (Heart Failure and Cardiac Regeneration) Research Group, Cardiology Service, University Hospital Germans Trias i Pujol, Crta. Canyet, s/n, 08916 Badalona, Barcelona, Spain; and Department of Medicine, Autonomous University Barcelona (UAB), Barcelona, Spain. abayesgenis@gmail.com

Complete recovery of ischemic cardiac muscle after myocardial infarction is still an unresolved concern. In recent years, intensive research efforts have focused on mimicking the physical and biological properties of myocardium for cardiac repair. Here we show how heart regeneration approaches have evolved from cell therapy to refined tissue engineering. Despite progressive improvements, the best cell type and delivery strategy are not well established. Our group has identified a new population of cardiac adipose tissue–derived progenitor cells with inherent cardiac and angiogenic potential that is a promising candidate for cell therapy to restore ischemic myocardium. We also describe results from three strategies for cell delivery into a murine model of myocardial infarction: intramyocardial injection, implantation of a fibrin patch loaded with cells, and an engineered bioimplant (a combination of chemically designed scaffold, peptide hydrogel, and cells); dual-labeling noninvasive bioluminescence imaging enables *in vivo* monitoring of cardiac-specific markers and cell survival.

Keywords: tissue engineering; cardiac regeneration; cardiac ATDPCs; noninvasive bioluminescence

Introduction

Heart failure of ischemic origin is the end stage of many cardiovascular diseases, such as acute myocardial infarction (AMI). AMI normally occurs when the blood supply to the heart is interrupted, leading to myocardial ischemia and necrosis following the formation of a large, noncontractile scar. Patients with enlarged hearts due to AMI suffer from progressive symptoms of heart failure and are at high risk of sudden cardiac death.[1] Therapeutic strategies that limit remodeling after heart failure may provide ways to reconstitute the affected tissue and function, recovering the structural support necessary for effective cardiomyocyte contraction. Currently, the only definitive treatment for heart failure is cardiac transplant, which is hampered in many instances by the limited number of heart donors and the process of graft rejection over time.

Cellular cardiomyoplasty

Cellular cardiomyoplasty is an alternative treatment currently under development. The objective of cellular cardiomyoplasty after AMI is to repair the damaged tissue by implantation of cardiomyogenic or angiogenic progenitor cells over the infarcted ventricle, with the expectation that engraftment of cells will contribute to the generation of new myocardial tissue and vessels.[2–5] One of the difficulties in cell-based strategies for restoring cardiac tissue relates to the optimum cell type. Despite the existence of resident cardiac stem cells,[6–9] the regenerative capacity of the adult heart is poor, motivating numerous research groups to seek the best source of cells with myocardial repair capacity.[10–13] Prior to clinical application, this optimal cell source must be able to be (1) expanded in large-scale *in vitro* culture, (2) engrafted within damaged tissue, and (3)

doi: 10.1111/j.1749-6632.2012.06519.x
Ann. N.Y. Acad. Sci. 1254 (2012) 57–65 © 2012 New York Academy of Sciences.

differentiated into new cardiac muscle cells that are electromechanically coupled with neighboring cells.[14] Various candidate cell types have been identified, such as adult stem or precursor cells from sources including bone marrow, adipose tissue, skeletal muscle, dental pulp, circulating blood, and joint synovium.[15–20] The autologous source of adult cells reduces concerns about immune rejection and disease transmission.

Embryonic stem cells have also garnered a great deal of attention. Although these cells are nonautologous, their pluripotent properties confer the ability to differentiate into myocytes, vascular cells, and cardiac fibroblasts, all of which are essential for full regeneration of the myocardium.[21–23] However, the undifferentiated state is associated with the risk of uncontrolled differentiation leading to teratoma formation.[24] To circumvent the nonautologous difficulty, two groups have developed induced pluripotent stem cells from somatic human tissues. Although these cells are autologous embryonic-like cells, the derivation of these cells involves the use of viral infection, which may activate oncogenes.[25–27] However, researchers are working on removing the oncogenes after the induction of pluripotency.[28,29] Alternatively, production of protein-induced pluripotent stem cells lacking genetic alteration has been achieved by treating the cells with polyarginin anchors to channel certain proteins through the cell membrane.[30]

In humans, several cell types, including bone marrow monocytes, myoblasts, and adult mesenchymal stem cells, have been delivered into the ischemic heart at various time-points and by different routes (intracoronary delivery, direct myocardial injection from the epicardium during open-heart surgery, or endomyocardial injection using specifically designed catheters). Taken together, these procedures show modest improvements in cardiac function and limited implanted cell survival in the fibrous myocardium. Neither interactions with preexisting cardiomyocytes nor electromechanical coupling through intercellular gap junctions have been reported, and cells do not withstand the mechanical forces and hypoxic conditions they experience in the host tissue.[4,31–36]

Tissue engineering for cardiac regeneration

The cell survival and implantation difficulties following cellular cardiomyoplasty have motivated the emergence in recent years of new approaches such as tissue engineering. Tissue engineering combines cells, biomaterials, and growth factors to generate functional three-dimensional tissue outside of the body that exhibits the required properties for the host tissue. Cardiac regeneration requires *in vitro* mimicry of the differentiated conditions of the heart at the molecular, structural, and functional levels to facilitate implantation and coupling of the bioengineered structure into the myocardium.

Experimental and clinical studies have been performed with regard to stem cell therapy as well as tissue-engineering approaches for myocardial support and regeneration. Examples include (1) implantation of scaffold-free cell sheets,[37,38] (2) direct injection of the biomaterial/cell mixture into the damaged tissue (*in situ* engineering),[39–41] and (3) implantation of biomaterial as a porous scaffold structure or a dense patch structure.[42–49] Based on composition, biomaterials can be divided into natural materials (extracellular matrix derivatives, alginate, fibrin glue), synthetic materials (polyesters, elastomeric polymers), or a combination of natural and synthetic materials, all with submicron pores and nanotopography surfaces.[4,43,50–52] Biomaterials should be able to circumvent cell retention and survival difficulties, entrapping cells *in situ* and allowing their customization by addition of prosurvival or growth factors that enhance the myogenic or angiogenic capacity of implanted cells while protecting them from the ischemic environment.[53–55]

Despite intensive efforts and initially encouraging results, cell survival and functionality of tissue-engineered cardiac implants remain poor. We are aware of these difficulties and are focused on identifying the most appropriate cellular type for myocardial repair and on developing new tissue engineering strategies for improving cell administration and survival in the necrotic myocardium.

Cardiac adipose tissue as a cell source for cellular cardiomyoplasty

In humans, cardiac adipose tissue is mainly found in the atrioventricular and interventricular grooves, around the aortic root, and along the main branches of the coronary arteries. This adipose tissue was initially considered to be a protective cushion for the heart, but subsequent investigation demonstrated that it is also a metabolically active organ that generates hormones, cytokines, and chemokines. These molecules modulate cardiac function and exert cardioprotective effects against ischemia, including attenuation of cardiomyocyte apoptosis and reduction in infarct size.[56,57] With this information in mind, our group examined the adipose tissue that surrounds the heart as a possible source of progenitor cells for cellular cardiomyoplasty, with the ultimate aim of restoring injured myocardium.

We recently identified and characterized a novel population of human adult progenitor cells derived from cardiac adipose tissue (cardiac ATDPCs). These cells presented similar surface antigen expression as bone marrow-derived mesenchymal stem cells but did not differentiate into adipocytes, indicating reduced pluripotency and commitment to specific lineages.[5,58] In the absence of external stimulation, cardiac ATDPCs showed high gene and protein expression of major cardiac proteins such as GATA-4, connexin-43, sarcomeric α-actinin, SERCA2, and β-myosin heavy chain. Interestingly, cardiac ATDPCs were able to activate the cardiomyogenic marker troponin I (cTnI) *de novo* when cells were cultured with neonatal rat cardiomyocytes or when ATDPCs were intramyocardially delivered to mouse and rat models of AMI (Fig. 1A). *In vivo* studies have shown that cardiac ATDPCs exert a beneficial effect when transplanted into the infarcted myocardium, including cardiac function improvement and reduction in infarct size. Taken together, these results indicate that, although cardiac ATDPCs are located in adipose tissue, they have an inherent cardiomyogenic phenotype and may participate in heart homeostasis, perhaps serving as a cell reservoir for myocardial tissue renovation.

Additionally, cardiac ATDPCs may present endothelial cell lineage properties, as evidenced by microarray analysis, functional angiogenic assays, and *in vivo* transplant experiments.[5] These cells secrete proangiogenic factors under hypoxic conditions, suggesting a paracrine effect that enhances local angiogenesis. In sum, our observations indicate that this novel progenitor cell type in human adult cardiac adipose tissue has both cardiac

and endothelial cell potential. Moreover, these cells are nonteratogenic and have immunosuppressive effects, making cardiac ATDPCs a promising, safe candidate for future use in cell therapies for cardiac regeneration.

Tissue engineering using biological patches

Despite the promise of cellular cardiomyoplasty with cardiac ATDPCs and other cell types, experiments have revealed a partial contribution to regeneration of the damaged myocardium.[3,47,59–63] Most of the implanted cells die soon after transplantation due to the adverse mechanical forces and the hypoxic conditions they encounter.[61] The low rate of cell survival in the fibrous myocardium and the low level of interaction between the surviving cells and the host tissue[53,61] diverted our efforts to the implementation of cell therapy through the fixation of cell-seeded matrices over the infarcted ventricle (Fig. 1B).

As a first approach, we used fibrin glue as a natural patch system. Fibrin, the active truncated form of fibrinogen, has been widely used in tissue engineering due to its ability to serve as a biological glue, holding cells together in site as well as stimulating angiogenesis.[64,65] Injection of cells with fibrin glue into infarcted rat hearts increased cell transplantation survival, decreased scar size, and increased vessel density in the damaged area.[40,66]

Taking into account these previous investigations and the importance of tracking cell survival and differentiation, we designed an *in vivo* experiment in which we used fibrin glue for cell implantation and a noninvasive bioluminescence imaging (BLI) system for cell detection in the mouse model of AMI. Due to the ability of visible-light photons to cross-live tissue, BLI allows real-time monitoring of the location, proliferation, and differentiation of luciferase-expressing cells in living tissues. By using tissue-specific promoters to regulate the expression of luciferase reporters introduced into living cells, changes in promoter activity translate into measurable changes in photon fluxes that correlate with transcriptional activity. The promoter of cTnI was selected as a marker to monitor cardiac differentiation, and the cytomegalovirus (CMV)-constitutive promoter was used for the detection of cell proliferation. Both promoters regulate the expression of chimeric photoproteins with two types of activities:

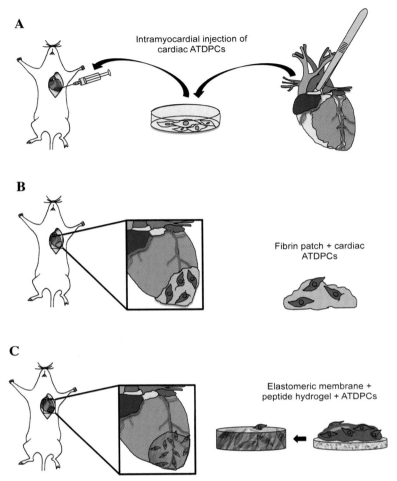

Figure 1. Schematic representation strategies for cell delivery into a murine model of myocardial infarction. (A) Intramyocardial cell injection. (B) Implantation of a fibrin patch loaded with cells. (C) Local delivery of an engineered bioimplant combination of a chemically designed scaffold, peptide hydrogel, and cells.

bioluminescence for noninvasive imaging, and fluorescence for histological analysis.[67]

For our study, cardiac ATDPCs were transduced with the lentiviral vectors CMV-RLuc-RFP-ttk (constitutive expression) and cTnIp-PLuc-eGFP (human-specific cTnI expression) (Fig. 2A). Once labeled, cells were loaded onto a three-dimensional fibrin patch and transplanted to cover injured myocardium in a severe combined immunodeficiency mouse model of myocardial infarction. Our goal was to monitor *in vivo* cTnI gene expression of cardiac ATDPCs via *in vivo* BLI. Light levels were quantified every week and animals were sacrificed at one month postimplantation. Initial BLI quantification indicated that *de novo* expression of cTnI

was already induced one week after cell implantation (Fig. 2B). cTnI expression was confirmed at the protein level by immunofluorescence (Fig. 2C). Despite the significance of cell differentiation in the host tissue, complete organ regeneration was not well achieved, suggesting the need for more sophisticated therapeutic platforms that limit the spread of the infarcted area and prevent excessive remodeling of the ventricle.

Bioengineered tissue implants for cardiac regeneration

We recently created a European consortium, Regeneration of Cardiac Tissue Assisted by Bioactive

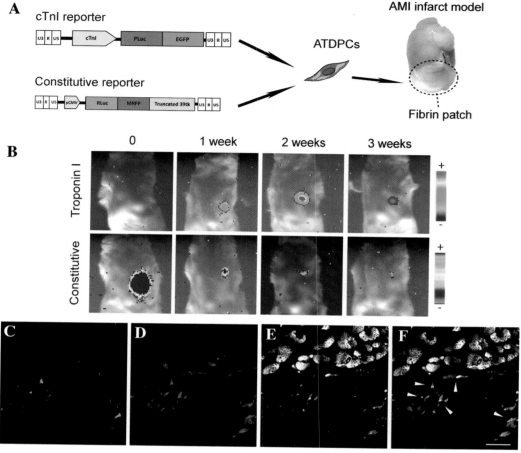

Figure 2. Fibrin patch approach for cardiac regeneration. (A) Diagram of the fibrin patch experimental design. Lentiviral constructs were employed as reporters for cell proliferation and cTnI differentiation. (B) Representative noninvasive BLI of dual-labeled cardiac ATDPCs within an implanted fibrin patch, regulated by a constitutive reporter (CMV:hRLuc:RFP:ttk) and a cell differentiation reporter (PLuc:eGFP) regulated by the cTnI promoter (hcTnIp). Luciferase images are superimposed on black and white dorsal images of the recipient animal. Color bars illustrate relative light intensities from PLuc and RLuc. (C–F) Immunofluorescence staining in mouse heart cross-sections transplanted with cardiac ATDPCs in a fibrin patch. Transplanted cells were detected with anti-RFP (red, D). cTnI expression was detected with anti-GFP (green, C) and anti-cTnI (white, E) antibodies; F is the merged image. Arrowheads indicate cTnI-expressing transplanted cells (colocalization). Nuclei were counterstained with Hoechst 33342. Scale bars: 25 μm.

Implants (RECATABI), with the objective of developing a bioengineered platform to generate novel bioimplants using innovative biomaterial combinations that will improve cell delivery, survival, migration, and differentiation into newly functional myocardial tissue. As a first approach, we tested a bioimplant consisting of scaffolds with interconnected spherical pores made of partially biodegradable polycaprolactone methacryloyloxyethyl ester or polycaprolactone methacryloyloxyethyl ester membrane loaded with peptide hydrogel (PuraMatrix™

BD Biosciences, Bedford, MA) and subcutaneous ATDPCs in the AMI murine model (Fig. 1C). Preliminary BLI quantification indicated a nice constitutive reporter signal postimplantation, and we were able to detect a progressive increase in cTnI expression in AMI and sham-operated animals (Fig. 3A). cTnI differentiation was confirmed at the protein level by immunofluorescence staining of cross-sectioned hearts. We therefore postulate that the cardiac environment, rather than signals coming from the injured area, exerts a differentiation

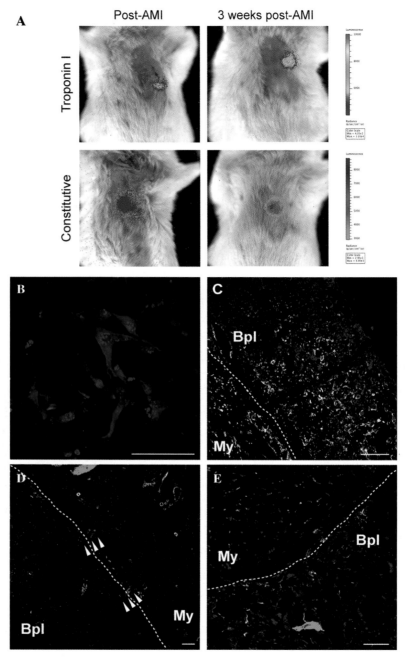

Figure 3. Engineered three-dimensional bioimplant for cardiac repair. (A) Representative noninvasive BLI of dual-labeled cardiac ATDPCs within a PCLMA and peptide hydrogel (bioimplant), regulated by a constitutive reporter (CMV:hRLuc:RFP:ttk) and a cell differentiation reporter (PLuc:eGFP) regulated by the cTnI promoter (hcTnIp). Luciferase images are superimposed on black and white dorsal images of the recipient animal. Color bars illustrate relative light intensities from PLuc and RLuc. (B) RFP constitutive expression in subcutaneous ATDPCs inside the bioimplant. (C–E) Immunofluorescence staining in mouse heart cross-sections transplanted with subcutaneous ATDPCs in the bioimplant (Bpl). Transplanted cells were detected with anti-RFP (red, B–E). Vessels were detected with isolectin staining (white, C–E) and FITC-dextran (green, D and E) for functionality. Arrowheads in D indicate vessels connecting myocardium (My) with the bioimplant. Nuclei were counterstained with Hoechst 33342. Scale bars: 50 μm.

effect over the implanted cells. Histological analysis also revealed the significant vascularization of the entire structure, which was connected to the myocardium (Fig. 3B–E). These observations indicate that not only is the bioimplant integrated into the myocardium, it also bears a portion of the human cells that can survive and modestly differentiate into cardiac-like cells.

Summary

We have reviewed various cell types and approaches underlying current efforts to regenerate the infarcted heart. Despite promising results in some studies, full recovery of injured myocardium and cardiac functions has yet to be achieved. Our group anticipates that cardiac adipose tissue will serve as an important source of progenitor cells with inherent cardiac and angiogenic potential. We are currently working on various strategies, ranging from the bare injection of cells inside the myocardium to the bioimplant, a sophisticated combination of chemically designed scaffold, peptide hydrogel, and ATDPCs. Introduction of BLI technology has also conferred a significant improvement in the tracking of cell survival and differentiation.

Acknowledgments

The authors wish to thank the consenting patients who made this study possible and the members of the Department of Cardiac Surgery for their collaboration in obtaining human samples. We are also grateful to Carolina Gálvez for her graphic art contribution. This work was supported by Ministerio de Ciencia e Innovación (SAF 2008-05144-C02-01 and SAF2009-07102), the European Commission 7th Framework Programme (RECATABI, NMP3-SL-2009-229239), Fundació La Marató de TV3 (080330), and Fundació Privada Daniel Bravo Andreu.

Conflicts of interest

The authors declare no conflicts of interest.

References

1. Olivetti, G. *et al.* 1991. Cellular basis of chronic ventricular remodeling after myocardial infarction in rats. *Circ. Res.* **68:** 856–869.
2. Orlic, D. *et al.* 2001. Bone marrow cells regenerate infarcted myocardium. *Nature.* **410:** 701–705.
3. Genovese, J. *et al.* 2007. Cell based approaches for myocardial regeneration and artificial myocardium. *Curr. Stem Cell Res. Ther.* **2:** 121–127.
4. Chachques, J.C. *et al.* 2009. Cardiomyoplasty: is it still a viable option in patients with end-stage heart failure? *Eur. J. Cardiothorac. Surg.* **35:** 201–203.
5. Bayes-Genis, A. *et al.* 2010. Human progenitor cells derived from cardiac adipose tissue ameliorate myocardial infarction in rodents. *J. Mol. Cell Cardiol.* **49:** 771–780.
6. Beltrami, A.P. *et al.* 2003. Adult cardiac stem cells are multipotent and support myocardial regeneration. *Cell* **114:** 763–776.
7. Oh, H. *et al.* 2003. Cardiac progenitor cells from adult myocardium: homing, differentiation, and fusion after infarction. *Proc. Natl. Acad. Sci. U.S.A.* **100:** 12313–12318.
8. Laugwitz, K.L. *et al.* 2005. Postnatal isl1? Cardioblasts enter fully differentiated cardiomyocyte lineages. *Nature* **433:** 647–653.
9. Smith, R.R. *et al.* 2007. Regenerative potential of cardiosphere-derived cells expanded from percutaneous endomyocardial biopsy specimens. *Circulation* **115:** 896–908.
10. Orlic, D, *et al.* 2001. Transplanted adult bone marrow cells repair myocardial infarcts in mice. *Ann. N.Y. Acad. Sci.* **938:** 221–229
11. Rangappa, S. *et al.* 2003. Transformation of adult mesenchymal stem cells isolated from the fatty tissue into cardiomyocytes. *Ann. Thorac. Surg.* **75:** 775–779.
12. Behfar A, *et al.* 2010. Guided cardiopoiesis enhances therapeutic benefit of bone marrow human mesenchymal stem cells in chronic myocardial infarction. *J. Am. Coll. Cardiol.* **56:** 721–734.
13. Roura, S. *et al.* 2010. Exposure to cardiomyogenic stimuli fails to transdifferentiate human umbilical cord blood-derived mesenchymal stem cells. *Basic Res. Cardiol.* **105:** 419–430.
14. Vunjak-Novakovic, G. *et al.* 2010. Challenges in cardiac tissue engineering. *Tissue. Eng. Part B Rev.* **16:** 169–187.
15. Gimble, J.M., A.J. Katz & B.A. Bunnell. 2007. Adipose-derived stem cells for regenerative medicine. *Circ. Res.* **100:** 1249–1260.
16. Passier, R., L.W. van Laake & C.L. Mummery. 2008. Stem-cell based therapy and lessons from the heart. *Nature* **453:** 322–329.
17. Miura, M. *et al.* 2003. SHED: stem cells from human exfoliated deciduous teeth. *Proc. Natl. Acad. Sci. U.S.A.* **100:** 5807–5812.
18. Gandia, C. *et al.* 2008. Human dental pulp stem cells improve left ventricular function, induce angiogenesis, and reduce infarct size in rats with acute myocardial infarction. *Stem Cells* **26:** 638–645.
19. Zhang, S. *et al.* 2004. Both cell fusion and transdifferentiation account for the transformation of human peripheral blood CD34-positive cells into cardiomyocytes in vivo. *Circulation* **110:** 3803–3807.
20. Pei, M., F. He & G. Vunjak-Novakovic. 2008. Synovium derived stem cell-based chondrogenesis. *Differentiation* **76:** 1044–1056.
21. Kehat, I. *et al.* 2004. Electromechanical integration of cardiomyocytes derived from human embryonic stem cells. *Nat. Biotechnol.* **22:** 1282–1289.

22. Yang, L. *et al.* 2008. Human cardiovascular progenitor cells develop from a KDR+ embryonic-stem-cellderived population. *Nature* **453:** 524–528.

23. Caspi, O. *et al.* 2007. Tissue engineering of vascularized cardiac muscle from human embryonic stem cells. *Circ. Res.* **100:** 263–272.

24. Cao, F. *et al.* 2007. Spatial and temporal kinetics of teratoma formation from murine embryonic stem cell transplantation. *Stem Cells Dev.* **16:** 883–891.

25. Takahashi, K. & S. Yamanaka. 2006. Induction of pluripotent stem cells from mouse embryonic and adult fibroblast cultures by defined factors. *Cell* **126:** 663–676.

26. Takahashi, K. *et al.* 2007. Induction of pluripotent stem cells from adult human fibroblasts by defined factors. *Cell* **131:** 861–872.

27. Yu, J. *et al.* 2007. Induced pluripotent stem cell lines derived from human somatic cells. *Science* **318:** 1917–1920.

28. Woltjen, K. *et al.* 2009. piggyBac transposition reprograms fibroblasts to induced pluripotent stem cells. *Nature* **458:** 766–770.

29. Ivics, Z. *et al.* 2009. Transposon-mediated genome manipulation in vertebrates. *Nat. Methods* **6:** 415–422.

30. Zhou, H. *et al.* 2009. Generation of induced pluripotent stem cells using recombinant proteins. *Cell Stem Cell* **4:** 381–384.

31. Assmus, B. *et al.* 2006. Transcoronary transplantation of progenitor cells after myocardial infarction. *N. Engl. J. Med.* **355:** 1222–1232.

32. Janssens, S. *et al.* 2006. Autologous bone marrow-derived stem-cell transfer in patients with ST-segment elevation myocardial infarction: double-blind, randomised controlled trial. *Lancet* **367:** 113–121.

33. Lunde, K. *et al.* 2006. Intracoronary injection of mononuclear bone marrow cells in acute myocardial infarction. *N. Engl. J. Med.* **355:** 1199–1209.

34. Schachinger, V. *et al.* 2006. Intracoronary bone marrow-derived progenitor cells in acute myocardial infarction. *N. Engl. J. Med.* **355:** 1210–1221.

35. Povsic, T.J. *et al.* 2011. A double-blind, randomized, controlled, multicenter study to assess the safety and cardiovascular effects of skeletal myoblast implantation by catheter delivery in patients with chronic heart failure after myocardial infarction. *Am. Heart J.* **162:** 654–662.

36. Amado, L.C. *et al.* 2005. Cardiac repair with intramyocardial injection of allogeneic mesenchymal stem cells after myocardial infarction. *Proc. Natl. Acad. Sci. U.S.A.* **102:** 11474–11479.

37. Shimizu, T. *et al.* 2002. Fabrication of pulsatile cardiac tissue grafts using a novel 3-dimensional cell sheet manipulation technique and temperature-responsive cell culture surfaces. *Circ. Res.* **90:** e40.

38. Masuda, S. *et al.* 2008. Cell sheet engineering for heart tissue repair. *Adv. Drug. Deliv. Rev.* **60:** 277–285.

39. Kofidis, T. *et al.* 2004. Injectable bioartificial myocardial tissue for large-scale intramural cell transfer and functional recovery of injured heart muscle. *J. Thorac. Cardiovasc. Surg.* **128:** 571–578.

40. Christman, K.L. *et al.* 2004. Fibrin glue alone and skeletal myoblasts in a fibrin scaffold preserve cardiac function after myocardial infarction. *Tissue Eng.* **10:** 403–409.

41. Tokunaga, M. *et al.* 2010. Implantation of cardiac progenitor cells using self-assembling peptide improves cardiac function after myocardial infarction. *J. Mol. Cell. Cardiol.* **49:** 972–983.

42. Li, R.K. *et al.* 1999. Survival and function of bioengineered cardiac grafts. *Circulation.* **100:** II63–II69.

43. Leor, J. *et al.* 2000. Bioengineered cardiac grafts: a new approach to repair the infarcted myocardium? *Circulation* **102:** III56–III61.

44. Vizzardi, E. *et al.* 2012. Stem cells and repair of the heart: cell-releasing epicardial scaffolds. *J. Cardiovasc. Surg.* (Torino). Jan 17. [Epub ahead of print].

45. Radisic, M. *et al.* 2005. Mathematical model of oxygen distribution in engineered cardiac tissue with parallel channel array perfused with culture medium containing oxygen carriers. *Am. J. Physiol. Heart Circ. Physiol.* **288:** H1278–H1289.

46. Radisic, M. *et al.* 2006. Biomimetic approach to cardiac tissue engineering: oxygen carriers and channeled scaffolds. *Tissue Eng.* **12:** 2077–2091.

47. Cortes-Morichetti, M. *et al.* 2007. Association between a cell-seeded collagen matrix and cellular cardiomyoplasty for myocardial support and regeneration. *Tissue Eng.* **13:** 2681–2687.

48. Chiu, L.L. *et al.* 2008. Biphasic electrical field stimulation AIDS in tissue engineering of multicell-type cardiac organoids. *Tissue Eng. Part A* **17:** 1465–1477.

49. Tandon, N., *et al.* 2009. Electrical stimulation systems for cardiac tissue engineering. *Nat. Protoc.* **4:** 155–173.

50. Radisic, M. *et al.* 2004. From the cover: functional assembly of engineered myocardium by electrical stimulation of cardiac myocytes cultured on scaffolds. *Proc. Natl. Acad. Sci. USA* **101:** 18129–18134.

51. Zimmermann, W.H. *et al.* 2002. Tissue engineering of a differentiated cardiac muscle construct. *Circ. Res.* **90:** 223–230.

52. Ott, H.C. *et al.* 2008. Perfusion-decellularized matrix: using nature's platform to engineer a bioartificial heart. *Nat. Med.* **14:** 213–221.

53. Chachques, J.C. *et al.* 2004. Angiogenic growth factors and/or cellular therapy for myocardial regeneration: a comparative study. *J. Thorac. Cardiovasc. Surg.* **128:** 245–253.

54. Laflamme, M.A. *et al.* 2007. Cardiomyocytes derived from human embryonic stem cells in pro-survival factors enhance function of infarcted rat hearts. *Nat. Biotechnol.* **25:** 1015–1024.

55. Ferreira, L.S. *et al.* 2007. Bioactive hydrogel scaffolds for controllable vascular differentiation of human embryonic stem cells. *Biomaterials* **28:** 2706–2717.

56. Ahima, R.S. & J.S. Flier. 2000. Adipose tissue as an endocrine organ. *Trends. Endocrinol. Metab.* **11:** 327–332.

57. Pezeshkian, M. *et al.* 2009. Fatty acid composition of epicardial and subcutaneous human adipose tissue. *Metab. Syndr. Relat. Disord.* **7:** 125–131.

58. Pittenger, M.F. *et al.* 1999. Multilineage potential of adult human mesenchymal stem cells. *Science* **284:** 143–147.

59. Zimmermann, W.H. *et al.* 2000. Three-dimensional engineered heart tissue from neonatal rat cardiac myocytes. *Biotechnol. Bioeng.* **68:** 106–114.

60. Patel, A.N. & J.A. Genovese. 2007. Stem cell therapy for the treatment of heart failure. *Curr. Opin. Cardiol.* **22:** 464–470.

61. Chachques, J.C. *et al.* 2008. A Myocardial Assistance by Grafting a New Bioartificial Upgraded Myocardium (MAG-NUM trial): clinical feasibility study. *Ann. Thorac. Surg.* **85:** 901–908.

62. Godier-Furnémont, A.F. *et al.* 2011. Composite scaffold provides a cell delivery platform for cardiovascular repair. *Proc. Natl. Acad. Sci. U.S.A.* **108:** 7974–7979.

63. Miyagawa, S. *et al.* 2011. Tissue-engineered cardiac constructs for cardiac repair. *Ann. Thorac. Surg.* **91:** 320–329.

64. Ahmed, T.A., E.V. Dare & M. Hincke. 2008. Fibrin: a versatile scaffold for tissue engineering applications. *Tissue. Eng. Part B Rev.* **14:** 199–215.

65. Leor, J., Y. Amsalem & S. Cohen. 2005. Cells, scaffolds, and molecules for myocardial tissue engineering. *Pharmacol. Ther.* **105:** 151–163.

66. Christman, K.L. *et al.* 2004. Injectable fibrin scaffold improves cell transplant survival, reduces infarct expansion, and induces neovasculature formation in ischemic myocardium. *J. Am. Coll. Cardiol.* **44:** 654–660.

67. Vilalta, M. *et al.* 2009. Dual luciferase labelling for non-invasive bioluminescence imaging of mesenchymal stromal cell chondrogenic differentiation in demineralized bone matrix scaffolds. *Biomaterials* **30:** 4986–4995.

Ann. N.Y. Acad. Sci. ISSN 0077-8923

ANNALS OF THE NEW YORK ACADEMY OF SCIENCES
Issue: *Evolving Challenges in Promoting Cardiovascular Health*

Umbilical cord blood for cardiovascular cell therapy: from promise to fact

Santiago Roura,[1] Josep-Maria Pujal,[1] and Antoni Bayes-Genis[1,2,3,4]

[1]ICREC Research Group, Health Sciences Research Institute Germans Trias i Pujol (IGTP), Barcelona, Spain. [2]Cardiology Service, University Hospital Germans Trias i Pujol, Barcelona, Spain. [3]Department of Medicine, Autonomous University Barcelona, Spain. [4]Biomedical Research Networking Center in Bioengineering, Biomaterials and Nanomedicine (CIBER-BBN), Spain

Address for correspondence: Antoni Bayes-Genis, M.D., Ph.D., FESC, ICREC (Heart Failure and Cardiac Regeneration) Research Group, Cardiology Service, University Hospital Germans Trias i Pujol, Crta. Canyet, s/n, 08916 Badalona, Barcelona, Spain. abayes.germanstrias@gencat.cat

Endothelial recovery and cell replacement are therapeutic challenges for cardiovascular medicine. Initially employed in the treatment of blood malignancies due to its high concentration of hematological precursors, umbilical cord blood (UCB) is now a non-controversial and accepted source of both hematopoietic and non-hematopoietic progenitors for a variety of emerging cell therapies in clinical trials. Here, we review the current therapeutic potential of UCB, focusing in recent evidence demonstrating the ability of UCB-derived mesenchymal stem cells to differentiate into the endothelial lineage and to develop new vasculature *in vivo*.

Keywords: cardiovascular diseases; umbilical cord blood; mesenchymal stem cell

Introduction

Endothelial recovery and cell replacement are paramount therapeutic challenges for cardiovascular regenerative medicine.[1] Beyond pharmacological or surgical intervention, stem cell–based therapies are promising for regenerating injured human tissues through the promotion of vascular growth and repair.[2] The acquisition of phenotypic and functional characteristics of the endothelial lineage has been reported for progenitor cells isolated from bone marrow[3,4] and adipose tissue.[5] Umbilical cord blood (UCB) is currently emerging as a valuable stem cell source.[6] The absence of ethical concerns and unlimited cell supply due to the continuous growth of the world population, which is expected to remain at a constant annual level of 134 million births according to U.S. Census Bureau estimations, explain the increasing interest in using UCB for a variety of clinical applications. In addition, UCB can be safely obtained and cryopreserved in either public or private banks without a loss of cell viability and has a lower risk of transmitting viral infections and somatic mutations than adult tissues.[7]

Here, we review the therapeutic potential of UCB in a spectrum of human disorders, including cardiovascular diseases, focusing on recent evidence that demonstrates the ability of UCB-derived mesenchymal stem cells (MSCs) to differentiate into the endothelial lineage and to develop new microvasculature *in vivo*.

Clinical applications of UCB

UCB was first employed as an alternative source of hematopoietic ($CD34^+$) progenitors in the treatment of autologous pediatric hematological malignancies.[8] Given that HLA-matching requirements for transplantation are not as strict as for other well-known hematopoietic stem cell sources, the use of UCB has been gaining acceptance for adult patients lacking matched (related or unrelated) bone marrow donors.[9] UCB is a noncontroversial and accepted stem cell source for cell therapy, and it has been extended to defective immune system reconstitution[10] and the correction of congenital hematological abnormalities.[11]

The most marked limitation in the use of UCB is its low progenitor cell concentration. Thus,

doi: 10.1111/j.1749-6632.2012.06515.x

ANNALS OF THE NEW YORK ACADEMY OF SCIENCES

Issue: *Evolving Challenges in Promoting Cardiovascular Health*

Heart repair: from natural mechanisms of cardiomyocyte production to the design of new cardiac therapies

Silvia Martin-Puig,[1] Valentín Fuster,[2,3] and Miguel Torres[1]

[1]Cardiovascular Development and Repair Department, [2]Epidemiology, Atherosclerosis and Imaging Department, Centro Nacional de Investigaciones, Cardiovasculares, Madrid, Spain. [3]Marie-Josée and Henry R. Kravis Center for Cardiovascular Health, Zena and Michael A. Wiener Cardiovascular Institute, Mount Sinai School of Medicine, New York, New York

Address for correspondence: Miguel Torres, Centro Nacional de Investigaciones Cardiovasculares, Instituto de Salud Carlos III, 3, Melchor Fernández Almagro, 28029 Madrid, Spain. mtorres@cnic.es

Most organs in mammals, including the heart, show a certain level of plasticity and repair ability during gestation. This plasticity is, however, compromised for many organs in adulthood, resulting in the inability to repair organ injury, including heart damage produced by acute or chronic ischemic conditions. In contrast, lower vertebrates, such as fish or amphibians, retain a striking regenerative ability during their entire life, being able to repair heart injuries. There is a great interest in understanding both the mechanisms that allow heart plasticity during mammalian fetal life and those that permit adult cardiac regeneration in zebrafish. Here, we revise strategies for cardiomyocyte production during development and in response to injury and discuss differential regeneration ability of teleosts and mammals. Understanding these mechanisms may allow establishing alternative therapeutic approaches to cope with heart failure in humans.

Keywords: heart development; cardiomyocyte generation; heart homeostasis; heart injury; cardiac regenerative therapies

The classical idea that the mammalian heart is a fully differentiated organ with no regenerative capacity is being revisited given several unexpected observations. It has been recently shown that human cardiomyocytes can slowly divide,[1] and an increasing amount of evidence points to the possibility that the mammalian heart may contain a resident progenitor population able to renew the adult myocardium.[2–7] Indeed, the mammalian heart displays after injury some of the tissular/cellular reactions typical of the cardiac regeneration process but in an inefficient way that cannot repair extensive cardiac damage. Unraveling the molecular mechanisms that govern cardiac development and regeneration could thus bring new information to the design of clinical strategies to enhance the limited regenerative capacity of the human heart in response to injury.

In this paper, we will review our current knowledge on heart development and regeneration in both mammals and fish, with a special focus on how the cardiomyocyte population is generated and maintained in various physiological and pathological situations. We will also review the various preclinical and clinical approaches that are being explored for heart repair in light of the accumulated knowledge on the mechanisms operating during heart development and regeneration.

Heart development

The heart is the first organ to form during vertebrate development and is essential for the distribution of nutrients and oxygen. Cardiogenesis is a morphologically complex process that implies sequential heart primordia migration, folding, looping, septation, and maturation to form the chambered heart. During this process, growth and differentiation of heart tissues have to be coordinated and tightly regulated in space and time.

Around the start of gastrulation in the mouse embryo, cardiac precursors in the epiblast move to the prospective anterior primitive streak[8] (Fig. 1A). At early gastrula, cardiac progenitors' ingress through

doi: 10.1111/j.1749-6632.2012.06488.x

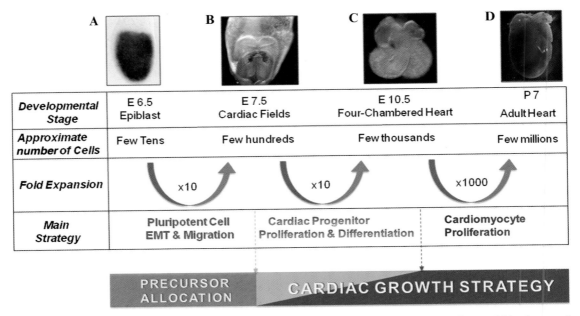

Developmental Stage	E 6.5 Epiblast	E 7.5 Cardiac Fields	E 10.5 Four-Chambered Heart	P 7 Adult Heart
Approximate number of Cells	Few Tens	Few hundreds	Few thousands	Few millions
Fold Expansion		×10	×10	×1000
Main Strategy		Pluripotent Cell EMT & Migration	Cardiac Progenitor Proliferation & Differentiation	Cardiomyocyte Proliferation

PRECURSOR ALLOCATION   CARDIAC GROWTH STRATEGY

Figure 1. Generation of cardiomyocytes during cardiogenesis. Top panels show representative pictures of sequential developmental stages of mouse embryo. (A) Oct4 *in situ* hybridization of an E6.5 embryo depicting the epiblast. (B) LacZ staining of an E7.5 embryo carrying the anterior heart field enhancer driving the expression of Cre recombinase (AHF-Cre) together with the Rosa26-LacZ activity reporter. ß-Galactosidase activity reveals SHF cardiac progenitors as a cardiac crescent, prior to their migration into the linear heart tube. (C) Bright field picture of an E10.5 embryo showing the looped heart with four chambers and outflow tract. (D) Bright field picture of a P7 mouse showing the four-chambered septated heart with aorta, pulmonary artery, and coronary arterial tree. The table indicates the approximate number of cardiac precursors or cardiomyocytes at each stage, the fold expansion, and the main strategy used for the generation of new cardiac cells. Note that as cardiogenesis progress, migration of pluripotent cells and proliferation plus differentiation of cardiac progenitors into the myocardium diminishes, and the main strategy to produce new cardiomyocytes becomes restricted to symmetric division from former cardiomyocytes. E, embryonic day; P, postnatal day; EMT, epithelial to mesenchymal transition.

the anterior primitive streak undergoing epithelial to mesenchymal transition (EMT) to form the cardiac mesoderm. These precursors then migrate anterior and laterally to position under the head folds, giving rise to the heart-forming regions (HFRs) with a characteristic cardiac crescent shape by E7.5 in the mouse embryo[9,10] (Fig. 1B). These committed progenitors, which express cardiac markers like Nkx2.5, Isl1, Gata4, or e/dHand, then swing toward ventral and medial to fuse at the midline, creating the linear heart tube by E8.0. The heart tube then experiences a rightward looping as early as E8.5, with the ventral side rotating and forming the outer curvature, whereas the dorsal part gives rise to the inner curvature. By E10.5, the shape of the heart is mostly defined, although there is not yet a proper septation of the chambers or the outflow tract[9,10] (Fig. 1C). The septation process is overall complete by

E14.5, and the heart shows a separation of the systemic and pulmonary circulation by connection of the left ventricle to the aorta and right ventricle to the pulmonary trunk, respectively. After septation, the heart continues growing its chambers while, in parallel, complex cell differentiation programs take place to generate the diversity of specialized cell types (e.g., pacemakers, smooth muscle cells, endothelial cells, interstitial fibroblasts, contracting myocardium, and conducting cells) that compose the mature heart[11] (Fig. 1D).

The primitive linear heart tube consists of just an inner layer of endothelial cells separated from the outer myocardial layer by a gelatinous material called cardiac jelly. The cardiac progenitors that generate this primitive heart tube are initially located in the most-lateral splanchnic mesoderm and are known as the first heart field (FHF) progenitors.

Once the primitive tube is formed, additional cardiac progenitors are added to the heart at both the arterial and the venous poles by migration from the mediocaudal splanchnic and pharyngeal mesoderm. These cardiac progenitors are thus known as second heart field (SHF) progenitors and have been identified in both chick and mouse by means of lineage tracing, genetic fate mapping, and retrospective clonal analysis.[12–19] SHF progenitors express the LIM-homeodomain transcription factor Isl1.[12,18,19] The discovery of the SHF allowed us to clarify the fate map of cardiac cells, according to which FHF progenitors give rise just to the left ventricular cardiomyocytes, whereas the SHF progenitors contribute to the entire right ventricle, part of the left ventricle, proximal outflow tract, and a significant amount of the atrial myocardium.[9,12,18,19] The picture may even become more complex with the recent discovery of cell type–specific early cardiac fields; a new endocardium-forming field has been identified medial to the cardiac crescent and incorporating to the heart tube through the arterial pole.[20]

In addition, further cardiac cell populations are added at later stages from various sources. Cardiac neural crest progenitors (CNCs) originate in the neural tube and migrate to the arterial pole of the heart through the pharyngeal arches. CNCs play a role in the remodeling of the outflow tract (OFT) and contribute to the smooth muscle cell layer of the aorticopulmonary septum and to the neurons and ganglia of the cardiac innervations.[21] Epicardial progenitors originate from splanchnic mesoderm and at early stages aggregate in the proepicardial organ (PEO), a structure lying adjacent to the sinus venosus. Afterwards, they migrate to the myocardium, forming the outer layer lining the heart, which is termed the epicardium.[22] Some of the epicardial cells undergo EMT and give rise to the epicardial-derived cells (EPDCs), which play a critical role on the formation of coronary vasculature, interstitial fibroblasts (reviewed in Ref. 22), and possibly to a small percentage of cardiomyocytes.[23,24]

Therefore, the current view proposes a model of progressive heart formation, with the participation not only of the FHF and subsequent addition of SHF precursors from cardiac mesoderm, but also of other sources of progenitors from outside the heart tube that contribute to different cardiac structures.[9,25]

Myocardium growth and maturation

Because myocardial mass loss and lack of contractility are the main causes of heart failure, there is a major interest in developing strategies to generate new cardiomyocytes. Thus, it is important to understand how cardiomyocytes are generated during heart development and regeneration and how this is maintained throughout adult life. The final adult myocardium structure and functionality is acquired through a series of maturational steps. Quantitative 3D reconstruction of cell proliferation patterns has allowed the defining of two strategies for the generation of cardiomyocytes[10,25–28] (Fig. 1B–D). Before primary tube formation, the cardiogenic mesodermal area proliferates very actively. As the FHF cells are added to the tube, they undergo drastic reduction in cell proliferation, in coincidence with their differentiation to cardiomyocytes. For the next few days, the SHF cells, still residing in the pharyngeal area, continue proliferating at a high rate to provide new cardiac precursors that will be added sequentially to both the arterial and venous poles of the heart tube. As SHF cells are added to the heart tube and begin to differentiate into cardiomyocytes, they again stop proliferation. The second strategy for cardiomyocyte proliferation starts around early looping stage and consists in the reactivation of cardiomyocyte cell cycle in the chamber-forming regions of the heart tube. Due to the sequential incorporation of precursors to the heart, the reactivation of cell proliferation in the prospective chambers overlaps in time with the proliferation of cardiac progenitors still in the SHF when the first cardiomyocytes added to the tube restart proliferation.

From E9.5 to E14.5, a subset of the compact layer cardiomyocytes migrates to the lumen, forming ridges first and finally finger-like projections, giving rise to the trabeculated myocardium. This type of myocardium is poorly proliferative and shows a more mature sarcomeric phenotype. Although arising from a common precursor, trabeculated and compact myocardium show obvious structural and proliferative differences and give rise to the ventricular conduction system and the compact working myocardium, respectively.[11] After septation of the chambers, the mammalian myocardium continues its maturational program and even at birth the sarcomeric structure is not fully organized, and only within early postnatal life the ventricular muscle acquires its characteristic rod shape and mature contractile apparatus.[29] It is at late prenatal or early postnatal stages when the growth of the heart switches from hyperplasia (growth by increasing the number of cells) to hypertrophy (growth by increase in size of existing cells), coinciding with the formation of binucleated cardiomyocytes.[30]

Therefore, new cardiomyocytes during development are first generated by migration and differentiation of cardiac precursors and afterwards by proliferation of cardiomyocytes (Fig. 1). Hence, there is a correlation between morphogenesis and heart proliferation that is further supported by the observation of differential gene expression regulating chamber formation (reviewed in Ref. 31). Notably, progenitor recruitment and differentiation is only used during a limited embryonic period and generates a limited number of cardiomyocytes, whereas the major part of the cardiomyocyte pool generation is achieved by symmetric division (Fig. 1). It is thus important to consider the molecular pathways involved in these transient proliferative episodes as well as the type of cardiomyocytes involved to design potential regenerative therapies.

Heart homeostasis

After birth, the mammalian heart undergoes a switch from hyperplasic to hypertrophic growth of myocardium. This process has been associated with the view of the heart muscle as a postmitotic organ and with the inability to recover the myocardial mass lost after an injury. Recent evidence, however, points to some ability of the mammalian heart to generate new cardiomyocytes. These new findings have fueled interest in exploring to what extent the adult cardiomyocyte population can be renewed by symmetric division or by differentiation of precursor cell populations. The recent demonstration of a modest but clear proliferation ability of human adult cardiomyocytes[1] has reactivated the hope for a potential therapy oriented to enhance this limited proliferative capacity. Bergmann and colleagues found a low division rate of 1% yearly in 25-year-old individuals but only 0.45% at the age of 75. According to their data, less than 50% of cardiomyocytes are generated by cell divisions taking place along the human lifespan. Interestingly, these results do not support the existence of a discrete pool of cardiomyocytes with differential turnover rate, but

rather suggest that all cardiomyocytes at a given age have similar chances to proliferate. Finally, the DNA carbon dating methodology used by the authors does not allow determining whether the new cardiomyocytes arise from preexisting cardiomyocytes or from a pool of stem/precursor cells. In this regard, a genetic fate-mapping study from Richard Lee's laboratory suggests that in the mouse there is no significant cardiomyocyte turnover sustained by a progenitor cell population in homeostatic conditions.[2] Interestingly, cardiomyocyte turnover was observed after myocardial infarction (MI) around the borders of the infarcted area. Nonetheless, these results were based on negative cell labeling and would require confirmation by a complementary positive-marking method that would identify the progenitor cell population responsible for the cardiomyocyte turnover.[2] In contrast to the limited cardiomyocyte renewal ability in mammals, heart homeostasis is effective throughout life in zebrafish via cardiomyocyte hyperplasia and epicardial signals.[32]

In summary, although there is evidence for limited proliferation and/or renewal of cardiomyoctes during mammalian heart homeostasis, direct *in vivo* evidence of a progenitor cell pool in charge of continuous cardiomyocyte generation has not been obtained.

Heart regeneration

Lower vertebrates, such as teleosts and amphibians, have a surprising ability to regenerate their myocardium during adult life.[33] Interestingly, recent studies in mice indicate that mammals retain a very similar ability but restricted to the first few days postbirth.[34] Investigating the mechanisms that allow this natural heart regeneration is of obvious interest for the design of heart repair strategies in humans. The zebrafish completely regenerates the myocardium within 60 days after resection of 20% of the ventricle by proliferation of cardiomyocytes. Interestingly, this process takes place without scar formation.[33] After myocardial damage, the epicardium responds by proliferation and reexpression of embryonic genes like *tbx18*, *wt1*, or *raldh2*.[35–38] Cardiac regeneration stimulates mobilization of EPDCs into the injured myocardium and their contribution to the generation of perivascular cells and fibroblasts improve cardiac recovery.[35,37] Despite the epicardial activation, there is no evidence that the production promising research area is the search for treatments that may stimulate CRPs cardiac repair potential.

Even though the field has been polarized in the search for CRPs and exogenous progenitor cells with *de novo* cardiogenic potential, the evidence from normal development and natural regeneration strategies in both mammals and fish is that the main strategy for increasing or recovering cardiomyocyte numbers is to stimulate their symmetric division. An important area of research directed to stimulate cardiomyocyte proliferation can be envisioned here in various directions. On the one hand, it will be illustrative to deeply characterize cellular and systemic differences of teleosts/mammalian neonates and adult mammals that may underlie their distinct regenerative capacities. On the other hand, it will be very interesting to explore treatments that may activate the proliferative response in adult cardiomyocytes. In this context, a potential therapeutic strategy could be based on gene therapy directed to cardiomyocytes. Clinical trials targeted to the SUMO-1/SERCA2a pathway using adeno-associated viral vectors have shown safe and beneficial effects on cardiac function and structure.[67,68] The combination of the advances in the field of cardiac gene therapy with those in cardiac regeneration may lead to promising future strategies to promote cardiomyocyte number recovery after MI.

A further tendency in the field is to eliminate the use of any virus- or cell-based strategy, as this may lead to easier treatments and more feasible clinical trials. Therefore, the stimulation of endogenous regenerative potential appears as a more attractive future approach. In this regard, it will be essential to characterize the secretome of endogenous (epicardium) or exogenous (BMCs) sources of regenerative signals. Identification of the *secreter* and *receiver* cells could identify candidate molecules to be used as soluble factors to potentiate regeneration. These strategies, however, will not be restricted to the use of classical drugs or signaling molecules, as the field of RNA and DNA molecules as therapeutic agents is rapidly evolving.

Finally, understanding tissue complexity will be essential to design proper therapeutic strategies. In this area, it will be important to define whether adult cardiomyocytes represent a heterogeneous population and how this relates to the differential proliferative or survival abilities in different species. If heterogeneous, how is the diversity generated/maintained? Is it associated to nuclear content, expression of certain receptors, or epigenetic and/or microenvironment regulation? The same case applies to the epicardium. Are the cells that secrete paracrine factors after MI the same that undergo EMT and differentiate into perivascular cells, or there are responder-only EPs that have a different cellular and molecular signature? Answering these important questions will significantly influence the improvement of cardiac regenerative therapies.

Acknowledgments

We thank Cristina Claveria for *in situ* hybridization of Oct4 and Juan Manuel Gonzalez-Rosa for software assistance. The Centro Nacional de Investigaciones Cardiovasculares is supported by the Spanish Ministry of Science and Innovation and the Pro-CNIC Foundation.

Conflicts of interest

The authors declare no conflicts of interest.

References

1. Bergmann, O. *et al.* 2009. Evidence for cardiomyocyte renewal in humans. *Science* **324:** 98–102.
2. Hsieh, P.C. *et al.* 2007. Evidence from a genetic fate-mapping study that stem cells refresh adult mammalian cardiomyocytes after injury. *Nat. Med.* **13:** 970–974.
3. Loffredo, F.S. *et al.* 2011. Bone marrow-derived cell therapy stimulates endogenous cardiomyocyte progenitors and promotes cardiac repair. *Cell Stem Cell* **8:** 389–398.
4. Smart, N. *et al.* 2011. De novo cardiomyocytes from within the activated adult heart after injury. *Nature* **474:** 640–644.
5. Laflamme, M.A. & C.E. Murry. 2011. Heart regeneration. *Nature* **473:** 326–335.
6. Chong, J.J. *et al.* 2011. Adult cardiac-resident MSC-like stem cells with a proepicardial origin. *Cell Stem Cell* **9:** 527–540.
7. Leri, A., J. Kajstura & P. Anversa. 2011. Role of cardiac stem cells in cardiac pathophysiology: a paradigm shift in human myocardial biology. *Circ. Res.* **109:** 941–961.
8. Nakajima, Y. 2010. Second lineage of heart forming region provides new understanding of conotruncal heart defects. *Congenit. Anom. (Kyoto)* **50:** 8–14.
9. Buckingham, M., S. Meilhac & S. Zaffran. 2005. Building the mammalian heart from two sources of myocardial cells. *Nat. Rev. Genet.* **6:** 826–835.
10. Aanhaanen, W.T. *et al.* 2012. Developmental origin, growth, and three-dimensional architecture of the atrioventricular conduction axis of the mouse heart. *Circ. Res.* **107:** 728–736.
11. Moorman, A.F., G. van den Berg, R.H. Anderson, V.M. Christoffels. 2010. Early cardiac growth and the ballooning model of cardiac chamber formation. In *Heart Development*

and *Regeneration*, Vol. 1. N. Rosenthal & R.P. Harvey, Eds.: 219–233. Elsevier. New York.

12. Cai, C.L. *et al.* 2003. Isl1 identifies a cardiac progenitor population that proliferates prior to differentiation and contributes a majority of cells to the heart. *Dev. Cell* **5:** 877–889.

13. Mjaatvedt, C.H. *et al.* 2001. The outflow tract of the heart is recruited from a novel heart-forming field. *Dev. Biol.* **238:** 97–109.

14. Waldo, K.L. *et al.* 2001. Conotruncal myocardium arises from a secondary heart field. *Development* **128:** 3179–3188.

15. Kelly, R.G., N.A. Brown & M.E. Buckingham. 2001. The arterial pole of the mouse heart forms from Fgf10-expressing cells in pharyngeal mesoderm. *Dev. Cell* **1:** 435–440.

16. Zaffran, S. *et al.* 2004. Right ventricular myocardium derives from the anterior heart field. *Circ. Res.* **95:** 261–268.

17. Meilhac, S.M. *et al.* 2004. The clonal origin of myocardial cells in different regions of the embryonic mouse heart. *Dev. Cell* **6:** 685–698.

18. Moretti, A. *et al.* 2006. Multipotent embryonic isl1⁺ progenitor cells lead to cardiac, smooth muscle, and endothelial cell diversification. *Cell* **127:** 1151–1165.

19. Sun, Y. *et al.* 2007. Islet 1 is expressed in distinct cardiovascular lineages, including pacemaker and coronary vascular cells. *Dev. Biol.* **304:** 286–296.

20. Milgrom-Hoffman, M. *et al.* 2011. The heart endocardium is derived from vascular endothelial progenitors. *Development* **138:** 4777–4787.

21. Snider, P. *et al.* 2007. Cardiovascular development and the colonizing cardiac neural crest lineage. *ScientificWorldJournal* **7:** 1090–1113.

22. Perez-Pomares, J.M. & J.L. de la Pompa. 2011. Signaling during epicardium and coronary vessel development. *Circ. Res.* **109:** 1429–1442.

23. Cai, C.L. *et al.* 2008. A myocardial lineage derives from Tbx18 epicardial cells. *Nature* **454:** 104–108.

24. Zhou, B. *et al.* 2008. Epicardial progenitors contribute to the cardiomyocyte lineage in the developing heart. *Nature* **454:** 109–113.

25. van den Berg, G. & A.F. Moorman. 2009. Concepts of cardiac development in retrospect. *Pediatr. Cardiol.* **30:** 580–587.

26. Soufan, A.T. *et al.* 2006. Regionalized sequence of myocardial cell growth and proliferation characterizes early chamber formation. *Circ. Res.* **99:** 545–552.

27. Sizarov, A. *et al.* 2011. Formation of the building plan of the human heart: morphogenesis, growth, and differentiation. *Circulation* **123:** 1125–1135.

28. de Boer, B.A. *et al.* 2011. The interactive presentation of 3D information obtained from reconstructed datasets and 3D placement of single histological sections with the 3D portable document format. *Development* **138:** 159–167.

29. Leu, M., E. Ehler & J.C. Perriard. 2001. Characterisation of postnatal growth of the murine heart. *Anat. Embryol. (Berl).* **204:** 217–224.

30. Porrello, E.R., R.E. Widdop & L.M. Delbridge. 2008. Early origins of cardiac hypertrophy: does cardiomyocyte attrition programme for pathological 'catch-up' growth of the heart? *Clin. Exp. Pharmacol. Physiol.* **35:** 1358–1364.

31. Risebro CA, R. P. 2006. Formation of the ventricles. *Scientific World Journal* **6:** 1862–1880.

32. Wills, A.A. *et al.* 2008. Regulated addition of new myocardial and epicardial cells fosters homeostatic cardiac growth and maintenance in adult zebrafish. *Development* **135:** 183–192.

33. Poss, K.D., L.G. Wilson & M.T. Keating. 2002. Heart regeneration in zebrafish. *Science* **298:** 2188–2190.

34. Porrello, E.R. *et al.* 2011. Transient regenerative potential of the neonatal mouse heart. *Science* **331:** 1078–1080.

35. Kikuchi, K. *et al.* 2011. tcf21⁺ epicardial cells adopt nonmyocardial fates during zebrafish heart development and regeneration. *Development.* **138:** 2895–2902.

36. Kikuchi, K. *et al.* 2011. Retinoic acid production by endocardium and epicardium is an injury response essential for zebrafish heart regeneration. *Dev. Cell* **20:** 397–404.

37. Lepilina, A. *et al.* 2006. A dynamic epicardial injury response supports progenitor cell activity during zebrafish heart regeneration. *Cell* **127:** 607–619.

38. Gonzalez-Rosa, J.M. *et al.* 2011. Extensive scar formation and regression during heart regeneration after cryoinjury in zebrafish. *Development* **138:** 1663–1674.

39. Jopling, C. *et al.* 2010. Zebrafish heart regeneration occurs by cardiomyocyte dedifferentiation and proliferation. *Nature* **464:** 606–609.

40. Kikuchi, K. *et al.* 2010. Primary contribution to zebrafish heart regeneration by gata4(+) cardiomyocytes. *Nature* **464:** 601–605.

41. Zhou, B. *et al.* 2011. Adult mouse epicardium modulates myocardial injury by secreting paracrine factors. *J. Clin. Invest.* **121:** 1894–1904.

42. Zhou, B. *et al.* 2012. Thymosin beta 4 treatment after myocardial infarction does not reprogram epicardial cells into cardiomyocytes. *J. Mol. Cell Cardiol.* **52:** 43–47.

43. Beltrami, A.P. *et al.* 2001. Evidence that human cardiac myocytes divide after myocardial infarction. *N. Engl. J. Med.* **344:** 1750–1757.

44. Drenckhahn, J.D. *et al.* 2008. Compensatory growth of healthy cardiac cells in the presence of diseased cells restores tissue homeostasis during heart development. *Dev. Cell* **15:** 521–533.

45. Li, F. *et al.* 1996. Rapid transition of cardiac myocytes from hyperplasia to hypertrophy during postnatal development. *J. Mol. Cell Cardiol.* **28:** 1737–1746.

46. Olivetti, G. *et al.* 1996. Acute myocardial infarction in humans is associated with activation of programmed myocyte cell death in the surviving portion of the heart. *J. Mol. Cell Cardiol.* **28:** 2005–2016.

47. Mercola, M., P. Ruiz-Lozano & M.D. Schneider. 2011. Cardiac muscle regeneration: lessons from development. *Genes Dev.* **25:** 299–309.

48. Mummery, C. & M.J. Goumans. 2011. Shedding new light on the mechanism underlying stem cell therapy for the heart. *Mol. Ther.* **19:** 1186–1188.

49. Martin-Puig, S., Z. Wang & K.R. Chien. 2008. Lives of a heart cell: tracing the origins of cardiac progenitors. *Cell Stem Cell* **2:** 320–331.

50. Bolli, R. *et al.* 2011. Cardiac stem cells in patients with ischaemic cardiomyopathy (SCIPIO): initial results of a randomised phase 1 trial. *Lancet* **378:** 1847–1857.

51. Pasumarthi, K.B. & L.J. Field. 2002. Cardiomyocyte cell cycle regulation. *Circ. Res.* **90:** 1044–1054.

52. Engel, F.B. *et al.* 2006. FGF1/p38 MAP kinase inhibitor therapy induces cardiomyocyte mitosis, reduces scarring, and rescues function after myocardial infarction. *Proc. Natl. Acad. Sci. USA.* **103:** 15546–15551.

53. Kuhn, B. *et al.* 2007. Periostin induces proliferation of differentiated cardiomyocytes and promotes cardiac repair. *Nat. Med.* **13:** 962–969.

54. Bersell, K. *et al.* 2009. Neuregulin1/ErbB4 signaling induces cardiomyocyte proliferation and repair of heart injury. *Cell* **138:** 257–270.

55. van Rooij, E., W.S. Marshall & E.N. Olson. 2008. Toward microRNA-based therapeutics for heart disease: the sense in antisense. *Circ. Res.* **103:** 919–928.

56. Hassink, R.J. *et al.* 2008. Cardiomyocyte cell cycle activation improves cardiac function after myocardial infarction. *Cardiovasc. Res.* **78:** 18–25.

57. Rasmussen, T.L. *et al.* 2011. Getting to the heart of myocardial stem cells and cell therapy. *Circulation* **123:** 1771–1779.

58. Williams, A.R. & J.M. Hare. 2011. Mesenchymal stem cells: biology, pathophysiology, translational findings, and therapeutic implications for cardiac disease. *Circ. Res.* **109:** 923–940.

59. Zaruba, M.M. *et al.* 2009. Synergy between CD26/DPP-IV inhibition and G-CSF improves cardiac function after acute myocardial infarction. *Cell Stem Cell* **4:** 313–323.

60. Davis, R.P. *et al.* 2011. Pluripotent stem cell models of cardiac disease and their implication for drug discovery and development. *Trends Mol. Med.* **17:** 475–484.

61. Zhao, T. *et al.* 2011. Immunogenicity of induced pluripotent stem cells. *Nature* **474:** 212–215.

62. Okita, K., N. Nagata & S. Yamanaka. 2011. Immunogenicity of induced pluripotent stem cells. *Circ. Res.* **109:** 720–721.

63. Elliott, D.A. *et al.* 2011. NKX2-5(eGFP/w) hESCs for isolation of human cardiac progenitors and cardiomyocytes. *Nat. Methods* **8:** 1037–1040.

64. Dubois, N.C. *et al.* 2011. SIRPA is a specific cell-surface marker for isolating cardiomyocytes derived from human pluripotent stem cells. *Nat. Biotechnol.* **29:** 1011–1018.

65. Ieda, M. *et al.* 2010. Direct reprogramming of fibroblasts into functional cardiomyocytes by defined factors. *Cell* **142:** 375–386.

66. Efe, J.A. *et al.* 2011. Conversion of mouse fibroblasts into cardiomyocytes using a direct reprogramming strategy. *Nat. Cell Biol.* **13:** 215–222.

67. Jessup, M. *et al.* 2011. Calcium Upregulation by Percutaneous Administration of Gene Therapy in Cardiac Disease (CUPID): a phase 2 trial of intracoronary gene therapy of sarcoplasmic reticulum Ca^{2+}-ATPase in patients with advanced heart failure. *Circulation* **124:** 304–313.

68. Kho, C. *et al.* 2011. SUMO1-dependent modulation of SERCA2a in heart failure. *Nature* **477:** 601–605.

Ann. N.Y. Acad. Sci. ISSN 0077-8923

ANNALS OF THE NEW YORK ACADEMY OF SCIENCES
Issue: *Evolving Challenges in Promoting Cardiovascular Health*

Energy metabolism plasticity enables stemness programs

Clifford D.L. Folmes, Timothy J. Nelson, Petras P. Dzeja, and Andre Terzic

Center for Regenerative Medicine, Marriott Heart Disease Research Program, Division of Cardiovascular Diseases, Departments of Medicine, Molecular Pharmacology and Experimental Therapeutics, and Medical Genetics, Mayo Clinic, Rochester, Minnesota

Address for correspondence: Andre Terzic, M.D., Ph.D., Center for Regenerative Medicine, Mayo Clinic, Stabile 5, 200 First Street SW, Rochester, MN 55905. terzic.andre@mayo.edu

Engineering pluripotency through nuclear reprogramming and directing stem cells into defined lineages underscores cell fate plasticity. Acquisition of and departure from stemness are governed by genetic and epigenetic controllers, with modulation of energy metabolism and associated signaling increasingly implicated in cell identity determination. Transition from oxidative metabolism, typical of somatic tissues, into glycolysis is a prerequisite to fuel-proficient reprogramming, directing a differentiated cytotype back to the pluripotent state. The glycolytic metabotype supports the anabolic and catabolic requirements of pluripotent cell homeostasis. Conversely, redirection of pluripotency into defined lineages requires mitochondrial biogenesis and maturation of efficient oxidative energy generation and distribution networks to match demands. The vital function of bioenergetics in regulating stemness and lineage specification implicates a broader role for metabolic reprogramming in cell fate decisions and determinations of tissue regenerative potential.

Keywords: bioenergetics; glycolysis; oxidative metabolism; regenerative medicine; induced pluripotent stem cells; embryonic stem cells; lineage specification

Regenerative medicine is poised to transform medical practice by providing the prospect of definitive solutions for patients with degenerative diseases, for which curative therapies are currently lacking.[1,2] With aging of the global population, chronic noncommunicable diseases—led by the surge in cardiovascular disorders—are a recognized emerging pandemic.[3,4] Expanding the reach of current state-of-the-art therapies, stem cell–based reconstructive strategies aim at repairing disease pathobiology and restoring organ function. Through cell engraftment, growth and lineage specification, and/or recruitment of innate repair mechanisms, regenerative medicine is primed to advance care beyond palliation for a range of diseases, including cardiovascular conditions.[5,6] To date, clinical experience relies on the use of adult stem cells, which reside in natural body compartments, including the blood, adipose tissue, and bone marrow, but are restricted in their capacity for spontaneous lineage specification.[7] Beyond use of stem cells in their native state, recent evidence indicates that lineage prespecification offers enhanced therapeutic benefit.[8,9] A case in point is cardiopoiesis, whereby guided specification of the stem cell–source has been demonstrated as advantageous in the setting of heart failure therapy.[10,11] In this context, deconvolution of cellular fate plasticity is a key strategy for advancing the applications of cell-based regenerative medicine.[12–14]

Cell fate redirection

Remarkably, stem cells are not the sole regenerative source. Indeed, redirection of somatic differentiated cells back to the pluripotent state and transdifferentiation into alternative specialized lineages has recently been reported.[15–17] Why a specialized cell would maintain the potential to reactivate gene programs typical of another cell type is unknown. Yet, the uncovered cellular plasticity would endow the body with an innate repair capacity, with important implications for regenerative medicine applications. Cell fate redirection is

doi: 10.1111/j.1749-6632.2012.06487.x

achieved by perturbing the expression of specific combinations of transcriptional regulators that are naturally dormant in differentiated populations. In this way, nuclear reprogramming by overexpression of primordial transcription factor cocktails is sufficient to reset the gene expression pattern and somatic epigenetic landscape to an embryonic-like state.[18–20] Such induced pluripotent stem (iPS) cells recapitulate many of the features of natural inner cell mass–derived embryonic stem cells (ESCs), including their ability to give rise to tissues of all lineages, which defines genuine pluripotency.[21–30] The broad applications of iPS cells range from diagnostic platforms to unravel individual variation in disease susceptibility to personalized biotherapeutics offering next generation tools for functional regeneration.[31,32]

Metabolism in cell fate decisions

Beyond manipulation of the genetic and epigenetic state, modulation of energy metabolism and metabolic signaling has been implicated in cell fate decisions.[33–35] Examination of cellular bioenergetics documents that modulation of mitochondrial infrastructure and metabolic pathways is vital for crosstalk with genetic programs ensuring direction of cell fate.[35,36] With emphasis on dedifferentiation of somatic cells back to the pluripotent ground state and subsequent redifferentiation into specific lineages, this cytotype interconversion implicates mitochondrial dynamics and energy metabolism as a rheostat-controlling cell identity (Fig. 1).

Metabolic control of dedifferentiation

Metamorphosis of metabolic infrastructure

Dedifferentiation of somatic cells back to the pluripotent ground state requires dramatic remodeling of the metabolic infrastructure to support the anabolic and catabolic requirements of pluripotent cells. Nuclear reprogramming induces a reduction in mitochondrial DNA (mtDNA), which results in diminished mitochondrial density compared to the parental somatic source, and similar to that observed in ESCs, the quintessential stemness archetype.[37–46] Mitochondrial localization also transitions during nuclear reprogramming from extensive cytoplasmic networks to a predominately embryonic perinuclear localization.[37,39,41,43,47–51] The perinuclear mitochondrial localization has been proposed to be a marker of stemness, as it is also observed in human hematopoietic and mesenchymal stem cells.[52,53] Remaining mitochondria undergo structural regression from mature mitochondria of somatic cells, characterized by branched and elongated structures with extensive intracellular membranes (cristae), to the predominantly spherical and cristae poor structures of iPS cells.[37,39,41–43]

Transcriptional profiling has revealed a significant remodeling of genes contributing to mitochondrial function and energy metabolism, with the upregulation of mitochondrial biogenesis genes during reprogramming, while expression of nuclear encoded mitochondrial genes remains constant.[37,54] A significant reconfiguration of glucose metabolism also occurs, with the upregulation of the initial and final steps of glycolysis and the nonoxidative branch

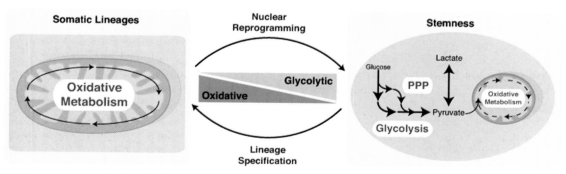

Figure 1. Energy metabolism plasticity regulates the balance between stem cell pluripotency and lineage specification. Somatic lineages efficiently generate ATP through complete oxidation of substrates in the mitochondria. In contrast, stem cells use glycolysis and the pentose phosphate pathway (PPP) to meet the anabolic and catabolic demands of stemness. The balance between glycolysis and oxidative metabolism contributes to the determination of cell fate, with nuclear reprogramming–induced mitochondrial regression and a greater reliance on glycolysis, while lineage specification results in mitochondrial biogenesis and the maturation of oxidative metabolism.

of the pentose phosphate pathway and downregulation of the intermediate reactions of glycolysis (*GPI, PFK,* and *ALDO*).[43,55] Bisulfite sequencing identified a large number of nuclear reprogramming–induced epigenetic modification of genes involved in glycolysis and oxidative metabolism.[56] In somatic cells undergoing reprogramming, upregulation of glycolytic genes precedes expression of pluripotent markers, suggesting a requirement for a metabolic switch in fueling reprogramming processes.[39] Transcriptional remodeling translates into a predominant downregulation of the subunits of the electron transport chain and upregulation of glycolytic enzymes in iPS cells, similar to that observed in ESCs.[39] Specifically, the isoform switch from hexokinase I to II and the upregulation of pyruvate dehydrogenase kinase—critical components at the mitochondrial–glycolysis interface—contribute significantly to induction of pluripotency, as inhibition of either of these targets reduces reprogramming efficiency.[39,43] Remodeling of the metabolic infrastructure is thus an essential and consistent attribute of nuclear reprogramming and supports the bioenergetic transition during pluripotent induction.

Metabolic switch defines pluripotency

Somatic cells completely oxidize metabolic substrates in the mitochondria to meet the energetic demands of cellular homeostasis. Nuclear reprogramming–induced regression of mitochondrial morphology would therefore suggest a significant impact on mitochondrial function. Pluripotent cells have elevated mitochondrial membrane potential compared to their parental somatic source, maintaining these cells in an energetically nascent, yet responsive state poised to meet the demands imposed by redifferentiation.[38,39,57] Direct assessment of mitochondrial oxidative competence indicates that pluripotent cells have reduced basal oxygen consumption and limited reserve capacity.[39,43] Although iPS cells have reduced energy turnover and total cellular adenosine triphosphate (ATP) levels compared to their parental sources,[37,39,42,43] the reduced oxidative capacity would require the use of alternative ATP-generating pathways to meet bioenergetic demands of self-renewal and proliferation. In this regard, recent metabolomics studies have indicated a bioenergetic switch from somatic oxidative metabolism to glycolysis during nuclear reprogramming (Fig. 1).[39,56] iPS cells have a

metabolome resembling that of ESCs but significantly different than parental cells, consistent with the upregulation of glycolysis, including elevated use of glucose and accumulation of lactate, and the downregulation of metabolites involved in tricarboxylic acid cycle and cellular respiration.[37,39,43,55,56] This observation is consistent across species and cell lines, indicating that the metabolic transition is a required marker of nuclear reprogramming success.[37,39,40,43,55]

Although the metabolome of iPS and ESCs are convergent, they are not necessarily identical, with iPS cells demonstrating lower abundance of unsaturated fatty acids and higher abundance of metabolites in the *S*-adenosyl methionine cycle.[56] High levels of unsaturated metabolites commonly found in ESCs are important for suppression of oxidative metabolism and maintenance of the pluripotent state, while *S*-adenosyl methionine is a key substrate for transmethylation reactions.[56,58] Indeed, supplementation with metabolites from either of these pathways significantly reduces nuclear reprogramming efficiency.[56] It remains unknown if other metabolic pathways that help to maintain pluripotency in ESCs, such as threonine metabolism and purine biosynthesis,[59] would significantly alter the efficiency of nuclear reprogramming.

Targeting energy metabolism for stemness induction

Energy metabolism is a novel target that can be manipulated to regulate the efficiency of nuclear reprogramming. Hypoxic stimulation of glycolytic flux improves the maintenance of stem cell pluripotency[60–63] and augments reprogramming efficiency.[64] Alternatively, inhibition of the p53 pathway, which in part stimulates glycolysis, also potentiates reprogramming.[65–70] Direct pharmacological modulation of energy metabolism or supplementation with glycolytic intermediates, accelerates glycolysis to augment reprogramming efficiency.[39,71] As proof of principle, agents that inhibit glycolysis and/or stimulate oxidative metabolism significantly suppress reprogramming efficiency.[39,71] The significance of optimizing energy metabolism during nuclear reprogramming is evidenced by the ability to reprogram cells with only a single stemness factor, OCT4, when glycolysis is stimulated in the presence of histone deacetylase, TGFβ, and MAPK/ERK inhibitors.[71] Therefore, a thorough understanding of the bioenergetic requirements of nuclear reprogramming, will allow for optimization of energy metabolism to promote pluripotency induction.

The glycolytic state in pluripotent cells may be required to fuel both catabolic and anabolic requirements.[33,72] Under the abundant supply of metabolic substrates in normal cell culture conditions, pluripotent cells may benefit from a faster rate of ATP generation from glycolysis, without being limited by the pathway's inefficient ATP generation.[33,35,73] Glycolysis in conjunction with the pentose phosphate pathway also provides a source of biosynthetic substrates and reducing cofactors that could match the anabolic requirements of cell proliferation. As the environment and complete oxidation of metabolic substrates cannot meet the demand for these cellular constituents, the glycolytic network can provide a capacity for generation and distribution of ATP and anabolic precursors to support cell proliferation and cellular homeostasis.[33,35,47,72] Anaerobicizing of somatic oxidative metabolism into pluripotent glycolysis thus fuels nuclear reprogramming and allows pluripotent cells to meet both anabolic and catabolic requirements.

Metabolic control of redifferentiation

Oxidative metabolism maturation fuels lineage specification

Remodeling of the mitochondrial and metabolic infrastructure matches the evolving bioenergetic requirements, as cells with a high energetic demand, such as the cardiomyocyte, drive the requirement for efficient oxidative ATP generation.[35,47,57] Spontaneous differentiation of stem cells is initiated by downregulation of pluripotent genes and the stimulation of mtDNA replication, which ultimately results in elevated mtDNA copy number to support mitochondrial biogenesis.[37,42,46,50,51,57,74] Concomitant to the increasing density of mitochondria is a maturation of their ultrastructure and localization to form networks of elongated and cristae-rich structures to allow energy transfer between specific cellular compartments.[37,42,47,50,51,57,75–77] Differentiation into lineages, especially those with high energetic demands, involves upregulation of tricarboxylic acid enzymes and electron transport chain subunits to support acceleration of cellular respiration and oxygen consumption to increase ATP produc-

tion.[47,50,57,74] Maturation of metabolic signaling and phosphotransfer infrastructure supports the glycolytic to oxidative metabolism transition in lineage specification (Fig. 1).[75,78] Neuronal and cardiac progeny derived from ESCs have a more saturated metabolome compared to their parental counterparts, consistent with a significant change in redox status during differentiation.[58] Treatment of ESCs with saturated substrates, including eicosanoids, saturated fatty acids, and acyl-carnitines promotes neuronal and cardiac differentiation.[58] Although these changes in bioenergetics coincide with differentiation of pluripotent cells, it remains unknown if a specific mitochondrial function and/or metabolic capacity must be obtained to overcome bioenergetic barriers and define specific lineages.

Metabolic markers of differentiation

The recent literature has demonstrated a growing role for mitochondrial dynamics and energy metabolism in driving pluripotent cell fate specification.[34,35,39] Inherent cell bioenergetic markers have been utilized to define the differentiation capacity of pluripotent cells. Despite these cells having similar expression of pluripotency markers and morphology, subsets of cells with less perinuclear localized mitochondria[79] and low-resting mitochondrial membrane potential have greater spontaneous differentiation.[80] Inhibition of maturation of the mitochondria and extended metabolic network inhibits differentiation,[57,78,81,82] although inhibition of the mammalian target of rapamycin, which significantly reduces mitochondrial oxygen consumption, increases mesodermal differentiation.[80] Mitochondrial content and function also defines the differentiation capacity of mesoangioblasts, a precommitted cardiac progenitor, with slow dividing cells, that contain abundant mitochondria with high membrane potential, efficiently differentiating into cardiomyocytes, while fast-dividing cells with few mitochondria do not respond to differentiation stimuli.[83] However, mitochondrial function may only be required during differentiation not for the maintenance of the progenitor state, as oxygen consumption is only elevated in the fast-dividing cells following induction of differentiation.[83] The differentiation block in fast-dividing mesoangioblasts can be reversed by increasing mitochondrial content, while loss of mitochondria in the slow-dividing cells impairs differentiation.[83] Mitochondrial dynamics also facilitate *in vivo* cardiac development as cardiomyocytes from early embryonic development contain few fragmented and immature mitochondria that transit into extensive networks of mature mitochondria in close proximity to the developing contractile filaments to ensure energetically competent development.[84]

Regulators of bioenergetic maturation

Some of the molecular components contributing to mitochondrial and bioenergetic maturation leading to pluripotent cell lineage specification have recently been elucidated. The mitochondrial permeability transition pore (mPTP), a non-selective conduit residing in the inner mitochondrial membrane has been identified as a gating mechanism underlying *in vivo* mitochondrial maturation and cardiomyocyte differentiation.[84,85] Early cardiomyocytes have a higher mPTP open probability, resulting in mitochondria with lower mitochondrial membrane potential and greater reactive oxygen species (ROS) generation, which ultimately impairs development.[84] Closure of mPTP facilitates maturation of mitochondria resulting in subsequent cardiomyocyte differentiation.[84] Additional regulators of permeability transition, including mitofusin-2, have been also implicated in pluripotent cell differentiation.[57,86] Permeability transition can affect cardiac differentiation via a number of vital downstream processes, including ROS production and energy metabolism. ROS flashes appear to modulate cardiomyocyte differentiation in both a time- and concentration-dependent fashion. Early commitment of cardiac progenitors may require ROS, with subsequent cardiomyocyte differentiation and maturation occurring under reduced ROS load, as addition of stable oxidants to immature cardiomyocytes impairs differentiation, while addition of antioxidants promotes cardiomyogenesis.[84,87,88] Low levels of ROS, potentially from high levels of glucose provided in cell culture, accelerate cardiac differentiation of stem cells by stimulation of cardiac genes and transcription factors,[89–92] while high levels of ROS appear to delay the process.[88,93] Transient mPTP opening also uncouples oxidative metabolism from ATP synthesis, which would maintain a high glycolytic capacity to support the immature state, while mPTP closure would promote oxidative metabolism to facilitate cardiac

differentiation.[34,35,85] This metabolic shift may also be regulated at the level of mitochondrial substrate supply, which is under the control of uncoupling protein 2 (UCP2).[94] Unlike UCP1, UCP2 has yet to display physiological uncoupling activity; however, it has been shown to suppress pyruvate oxidation and increase fatty acid and glutamine oxidation.[95–97] Owing to UCP2 expression in, predominately, glycolytic tissues and cancer cells and its ability to block mitochondrial pyruvate entry, UCP2 may promote glycolytic glucose use.[94,98–100] Indeed, gene silencing of UCP2 in pluripotent cells significantly reduces extracellular acidification rate (a surrogate marker of glycolysis) and ATP levels.[94] In contrast, UCP2 expression is reduced during differentiation of pluripotent cells, with ectopic expression of UCP2 both impairing oxygen consumption and pluripotent cell differentiation by blocking the metabolic shift from glycolysis to oxidative metabolism.[94] Taken together, maturation of mitochondrial function and energy metabolism is an essential component of pluripotent cell differentiation; however, further examination is required to define the intimate metabolic reprogramming conditions that drive the specification of diverse cell lineages.

Conclusion

Recent evidence has revealed a previously unrecognized role for energy metabolism in controlling the balance between maintenance of stemness and differentiation into specific lineages. The reliance on glycolysis has been documented to fuel the anabolic and catabolic requirements to maintain stem cells in the pluripotent state, while mitochondrial biogenesis and maturation of mitochondrial oxidative metabolism appears integral to match the energetic demands of differentiation. An enabling role for metabolic reprogramming in cell fate decisions offers a novel perspective on molecular events managing cell identity.

Acknowledgments

The authors are supported by the National Institutes of Health, the Canadian Institutes of Health Research, the Marriott Foundation, and the Mayo Clinic.

Conflicts of interest

The authors declare no conflicts of interest.

References

1. Terzic, A. *et al.* 2011. Regenerative medicine: on the vanguard of health care. *Mayo Clin. Proc.* **86:** 600–602.

2. Terzic, A. & T.J. Nelson. 2010. Regenerative medicine advancing health care 2020. *J. Am. Coll. Cardiol.* **55:** 2254–2257.

3. Terzic, A. & S. Waldman. 2011. Chronic diseases: the emerging pandemic. *Clin Transl. Sci.* **4:** 225–226.

4. Waldman, S.A. & A. Terzic. 2011. Cardiovascular health: the global challenge. *Clin. Pharmacol. Ther.* **90:** 483–485.

5. Nelson, T.J. *et al.* 2009. Stem cell platforms for regenerative medicine. *Clin Transl. Sci.* **2:** 222–227.

6. Bartunek, J. *et al.* 2010. Cells as biologics for cardiac repair in ischaemic heart failure. *Heart* **96:** 792–800.

7. Gersh, B.J. *et al.* 2009. Cardiac cell repair therapy: a clinical perspective. *Mayo Clin. Proc.* **84:** 876–892.

8. Behfar, A. & A. Terzic. 2006. Derivation of a cardiopoietic population from human mesenchymal stem cells yields cardiac progeny. *Nat. Clin. Pract. Cardiovasc. Med.* **3**(Suppl. 1): S78–S82.

9. Behfar, A. *et al.* 2008. Guided stem cell cardiopoiesis: discovery and translation. *J. Mol. Cell. Cardiol.* **45:** 523–529.

10. Behfar, A. *et al.* 2010. Guided cardiopoiesis enhances therapeutic benefit of bone marrow human mesenchymal stem cells in chronic myocardial infarction. *J. Am. Coll. Cardiol.* **56:** 721–734.

11. Marban, E. & K. Malliaras. 2010. Boot camp for mesenchymal stem cells. *J. Am. Coll. Cardiol.* **56:** 735–737.

12. Yamanaka, S. & H.M. Blau. 2010. Nuclear reprogramming to a pluripotent state by three approaches. *Nature* **465:** 704–712.

13. Mercola, M., P. Ruiz-Lozano & M.D. Schneider. 2011. Cardiac muscle regeneration: lessons from development. *Genes Dev.* **25:** 299–309.

14. Malliaras, K., M. Kreke & E. Marban. 2011. The stuttering progress of cell therapy for heart disease. *Clin. Pharmacol. Ther.* **90:** 532–541.

15. Takahashi, K. & S. Yamanaka. 2006. Induction of pluripotent stem cells from mouse embryonic and adult fibroblast cultures by defined factors. *Cell.* **126:** 663–676.

16. Jopling, C., S. Boue & J.C. Izpisua Belmonte. 2011. Dedifferentiation, transdifferentiation and reprogramming: three routes to regeneration. *Nat. Rev. Mol. Cell Biol.* **12:** 79–89.

17. Hussein, S.M., K. Nagy & A. Nagy. 2011. Human induced pluripotent stem cells: the past, present, and future. *Clin. Pharmacol. Ther.* **89:** 741–745.

18. Yu, J. *et al.* 2007. Induced pluripotent stem cell lines derived from human somatic cells. *Science* **318:** 1917–1920.

19. Wernig, M. *et al.* 2007. In vitro reprogramming of fibroblasts into a pluripotent ES-cell-like state. *Nature* **448:** 318–324.

20. Hochedlinger, K. & K. Plath. 2009. Epigenetic reprogramming and induced pluripotency. *Development* **136:** 509–523.

21. Lowry, W.E. *et al.* 2008. Generation of human induced pluripotent stem cells from dermal fibroblasts. *Proc. Natl. Acad. Sci. USA* **105:** 2883–2888.

22. Mikkelsen, T.S. *et al.* 2008. Dissecting direct reprogramming through integrative genomic analysis. *Nature* **454:** 49–55.

23. Meissner, A., M. Wernig & R. Jaenisch. 2007. Direct reprogramming of genetically unmodified fibroblasts into pluripotent stem cells. *Nat. Biotechnol.* **25:** 1177–1181.

24. Okita, K., T. Ichisaka & S. Yamanaka. 2007. Generation of germline-competent induced pluripotent stem cells. *Nature* **448:** 313–317.

25. Maherali, N. & K. Hochedlinger. 2008. Guidelines and techniques for the generation of induced pluripotent stem cells. *Cell. Stem Cell.* **3:** 595–605.

26. Martinez-Fernandez, A. *et al.* 2009. iPS programmed without c-MYC yield proficient cardiogenesis for functional heart chimerism. *Circ. Res.* **105:** 648–656.

27. Nelson, T.J. *et al.* 2009. Repair of acute myocardial infarction by human stemness factors induced pluripotent stem cells. *Circulation* **120:** 408–416.

28. Wernig, M. *et al.* 2008. Neurons derived from reprogrammed fibroblasts functionally integrate into the fetal brain and improve symptoms of rats with Parkinson's disease. *Proc. Natl. Acad. Sci. USA* **105:** 5856–5861.

29. Nelson, T.J. *et al.* 2009. Induced pluripotent reprogramming from promiscuous human stemness-related factors. *Clin. Transl. Sci.* **2:** 118–126.

30. Nelson, T.J., A. Martinez-Fernandez & A. Terzic. 2010. Induced pluripotent stem cells: developmental biology to regenerative medicine. *Nat. Rev. Cardiol.* **7:** 700–710.

31. Nelson, T.J. & A. Terzic. 2011. Induced pluripotent stem cells: an emerging theranostics platform. *Clin. Pharmacol. Ther.* **89:** 648–650.

32. Inoue, H. & S. Yamanaka. 2011. The use of induced pluripotent stem cells in drug development. *Clin. Pharmacol. Ther.* **89:** 655–661.

33. Vander Heiden, M.G., L.C. Cantley & C.B. Thompson. 2009. Understanding the Warburg effect: the metabolic requirements of cell proliferation. *Science* **324:** 1029–1033.

34. Folmes, C.D. *et al.* 2012. Mitochondria in control of cell fate. *Circ. Res.* **110:**526–529.

35. Folmes, C.D., T.J. Nelson & A. Terzic. 2011. Energy metabolism in nuclear reprogramming. *Biomark Med.* **5:** 715–729.

36. Breakthrough of the year: areas to watch. *Science* **334:** 1630–1631. www.sciencemag. org/content/334/6063/1630. full#named-content-3. Assessed January 30, 2012.

37. Prigione, A. *et al.* 2010. The senescence-related mitochondrial/oxidative stress pathway is repressed in human induced pluripotent stem cells. *Stem Cells* **28:** 721–733.

38. Armstrong, L. *et al.* 2010. Human induced pluripotent stem cell lines show similar stress defence mechanisms and mitochondrial regulation to human embryonic stem cells. *Stem Cells* **28:** 661–673.

39. Folmes, C.D. *et al.* 2011. Somatic oxidative bioenergetics transitions into pluripotency-dependent glycolysis to facilitate nuclear reprogramming. *Cell Metab.* **14:** 264–271.

40. Panopoulos, A.D. & J.C.I. Belmonte. 2011. Anaerobicizing into pluripotency. *Cell Metab.* **14:** 143–144.

41. Zeuschner, D. *et al.* 2010. Induced pluripotent stem cells at nanoscale. *Stem Cells Dev.* **19:** 615–620.

42. Suhr, S.T. *et al.* 2010. Mitochondrial rejuvenation after induced pluripotency. *PLoS One* **5:** e14095.

43. Varum, S. *et al.* 2011. Energy metabolism in human pluripotent stem cells and their differentiated counterparts. *PLoS One* **6:** e20914.

44. Lonergan, T., B. Bavister & C. Brenner. 2007. Mitochondria in stem cells. *Mitochondrion* **7:** 289–296.

45. Rehman, J. 2010. Empowering self-renewal and differentiation: the role of mitochondria in stem cells. *J Mol Med (Berl)* **88:** 981–986.

46. Facucho-Oliveira, J.M. & J.C. St John. 2009. The relationship between pluripotency and mitochondrial DNA proliferation during early embryo development and embryonic stem cell differentiation. *Stem Cell Rev Rep.* **5:** 140–158.

47. Chung, S. *et al.* 2010. Glycolytic network restructuring integral to the energetics of embryonic stem cell cardiac differentiation. *J. Mol. Cell. Cardiol.* **48:** 725–734.

48. Baharvand, H. & K.I. Matthaei. 2003. The ultrastructure of mouse embryonic stem cells. *Reprod. Biomed. Online* **7:** 330–335.

49. Baharvand, H. *et al.* 2006. Ultrastructural comparison of developing mouse embryonic stem cell- and in vivo-derived cardiomyocytes. *Cell Biol. Int.* **30:** 800–807.

50. Cho, Y.M. *et al.* 2006. Dynamic changes in mitochondrial biogenesis and antioxidant enzymes during the spontaneous differentiation of human embryonic stem cells. *Biochem. Biophys. Res. Commun.* **348:** 1472–1478.

51. St John, J.C. *et al.* 2005. The expression of mitochondrial DNA transcription factors during early cardiomyocyte in vitro differentiation from human embryonic stem cells. *Cloning Stem Cells* **7:** 141–153.

52. Piccoli, C. *et al.* 2005. Characterization of mitochondrial and extra-mitochondrial oxygen consuming reactions in human hematopoietic stem cells. Novel evidence of the occurrence of NAD(P)H oxidase activity. *J. Biol. Chem.* **280:** 26467–26476.

53. Chen, C.T. *et al.* 2008. Coordinated changes of mitochondrial biogenesis and antioxidant enzymes during osteogenic differentiation of human mesenchymal stem cells. *Stem Cells* **26:** 960–968.

54. Prigione, A. & J. Adjaye. 2010. Modulation of mitochondrial biogenesis and bioenergetic metabolism upon in vitro and in vivo differentiation of human ES and iPS cells. *Int. J. Dev. Biol.* **54:** 1729–1741.

55. Prigione, A. *et al.* 2011. Human induced pluripotent stem cells harbor homoplasmic and heteroplasmic mitochondrial DNA mutations while maintaining human embryonic stem cell-like metabolic reprogramming. *Stem Cells* **29:** 1338–1348.

56. Panopoulos, A.D. *et al.* 2012. The metabolome of induced pluripotent stem cells reveals metabolic changes occurring in somatic cell reprogramming. *Cell Res.* **22:** 168–177.

57. Chung, S. *et al.* 2007. Mitochondrial oxidative metabolism is required for the cardiac differentiation of stem cells. *Nat. Clin. Pract. Cardiovasc. Med.* **4**(Suppl. 1): S60–S67.

58. Yanes, O. *et al.* 2010. Metabolic oxidation regulates embryonic stem cell differentiation. *Nat. Chem. Biol.* **6:** 411–417.

59. Wang, J. *et al.* 2009. Dependence of mouse embryonic stem cells on threonine catabolism. *Science* **325:** 435–439.

60. Ezashi, T., P. Das & R.M. Roberts. 2005. Low O2 tensions and the prevention of differentiation of hES cells. *Proc. Natl. Acad. Sci. USA* **102:** 4783–4788.

61. Powers, D.E. *et al.* 2008. Effects of oxygen on mouse embryonic stem cell growth, phenotype retention, and cellular energetics. *Biotechnol. Bioeng.* **101:** 241–254.

62. Westfall, S.D. *et al.* 2008. Identification of oxygen-sensitive transcriptional programs in human embryonic stem cells. *Stem Cells Dev.* **17:** 869–881.

63. Mohyeldin, A., T. Garzon-Muvdi & A. Quinones-Hinojosa. 2010. Oxygen in stem cell biology: a critical component of the stem cell niche. *Cell Stem Cell* **7:** 150–161.

64. Yoshida, Y. *et al.* 2009. Hypoxia enhances the generation of induced pluripotent stem cells. *Cell Stem Cell* **5:** 237–241.

65. Bensaad, K. *et al.* 2006. TIGAR, a p53-inducible regulator of glycolysis and apoptosis. *Cell* **126:** 107–120.

66. Banito, A. *et al.* 2009. Senescence impairs successful reprogramming to pluripotent stem cells. *Genes Dev.* **23:** 2134–2139.

67. Hong, H. *et al.* 2009. Suppression of induced pluripotent stem cell generation by the p53-p21 pathway. *Nature* **460:** 1132–1135.

68. Kawamura, T. *et al.* 2009. Linking the p53 tumour suppressor pathway to somatic cell reprogramming. *Nature* **460:** 1140–1144.

69. Li, H. *et al.* 2009. The Ink4/Arf locus is a barrier for iPS cell reprogramming. *Nature* **460:** 1136–1139.

70. Marion, R.M. *et al.* 2009. A p53-mediated DNA damage response limits reprogramming to ensure iPS cell genomic integrity. *Nature* **460:** 1149–1153.

71. Zhu, S. *et al.* 2010. Reprogramming of human primary somatic cells by OCT4 and chemical compounds. *Cell Stem Cell* **7:** 651–655.

72. DeBerardinis, R.J. *et al.* 2008. The biology of cancer: metabolic reprogramming fuels cell growth and proliferation. *Cell Metab.* **7:** 11–20.

73. Pfeiffer, T., S. Schuster & S. Bonhoeffer. 2001. Cooperation and competition in the evolution of ATP-producing pathways. *Science* **292:** 504–507.

74. Facucho-Oliveira, J.M. *et al.* 2007. Mitochondrial DNA replication during differentiation of murine embryonic stem cells. *J. Cell Sci.* **120:** 4025–4034.

75. Chung, S. *et al.* 2008. Developmental restructuring of the creatine kinase system integrates mitochondrial energetics with stem cell cardiogenesis. *Ann. N. Y. Acad. Sci.* **1147:** 254–263.

76. Perez-Terzic, C. *et al.* 2003. Structural adaptation of the nuclear pore complex in stem cell-derived cardiomyocytes. *Circ. Res.* **92:** 444–452.

77. Perez-Terzic, C. *et al.* 2007. Stem cells transform into a cardiac phenotype with remodeling of the nuclear transport machinery. *Nat. Clin. Pract. Cardiovasc. Med.* **4**(Suppl. 1): S68–S76.

78. Dzeja, P.P. *et al.* 2011. Developmental enhancement of adenylate kinase-AMPK metabolic signaling axis supports stem cell cardiac differentiation. *PLoS One* **6:** e19300.

79. Lonergan, T., C. Brenner & B. Bavister. 2006. Differentiation-related changes in mitochondrial proper-

ties as indicators of stem cell competence. *J. Cell. Physiol.* **208**: 149–153.

80. Schieke, S.M. *et al.* 2008. Mitochondrial metabolism modulates differentiation and teratoma formation capacity in mouse embryonic stem cells. *J. Biol. Chem.* **283**: 28506–28512.

81. Varum, S. *et al.* 2009. Enhancement of human embryonic stem cell pluripotency through inhibition of the mitochondrial respiratory chain. *Stem Cell Res.* **3**: 142–156.

82. Spitkovsky, D. *et al.* 2004. Activity of complex III of the mitochondrial electron transport chain is essential for early heart muscle cell differentiation. *FASEB J.* **18**: 1300–1302.

83. San Martin, N. *et al.* 2011. Mitochondria determine the differentiation potential of cardiac mesoangioblasts. *Stem Cells* **29**: 1064–1074.

84. Hom, J.R. *et al.* 2011. The permeability transition pore controls cardiac mitochondrial maturation and myocyte differentiation. *Dev. Cell.* **21**: 469–478.

85. Halestrap, A.P. & P. Pasdois. 2009. The role of the mitochondrial permeability transition pore in heart disease. *Biochim. Biophys. Acta.* **1787**: 1402–1415.

86. Papanicolaou, K.N. *et al.* 2011. Mitofusin-2 maintains mitochondrial structure and contributes to stress-induced permeability transition in cardiac myocytes. *Mol. Cell. Biol.* **31**: 1309–1328.

87. Drenckhahn, J.D. 2011. Heart development: mitochondria in command of cardiomyocyte differentiation. *Dev. Cell.* **21**: 392–393.

88. Puceat, M. *et al.* 2003. A dual role of the GTPase Rac in cardiac differentiation of stem cells. *Mol. Biol. Cell.* **14**: 2781–2792.

89. Puceat, M. 2005. Role of Rac-GTPase and reactive oxygen species in cardiac differentiation of stem cells. *Antioxid. Redox. Signal* **7**: 1435–1439.

90. Sauer, H. *et al.* 1999. Effects of electrical fields on cardiomyocyte differentiation of embryonic stem cells. *J. Cell. Biochem.* **75**: 710–723.

91. Buggisch, M. *et al.* 2007. Stimulation of ES-cell-derived cardiomyogenesis and neonatal cardiac cell proliferation by reactive oxygen species and NADPH oxidase. *J. Cell Sci.* **120**: 885–894.

92. Crespo, F.L. *et al.* 2010. Mitochondrial reactive oxygen species mediate cardiomyocyte formation from embryonic stem cells in high glucose. *Stem Cells* **28**: 1132–1142.

93. Na, L. *et al.* 2003. Anticonvulsant valproic acid inhibits cardiomyocyte differentiation of embryonic stem cells by increasing intracellular levels of reactive oxygen species. *Birt. Defects Res. A. Clin. Mol. Teratol.* **67**: 174–180.

94. Zhang, J. *et al.* 2011. UCP2 regulates energy metabolism and differentiation potential of human pluripotent stem cells. *EMBO J.* **30**: 4860–4873.

95. Couplan, E. *et al.* 2002. No evidence for a basal, retinoic, or superoxide-induced uncoupling activity of the uncoupling protein 2 present in spleen or lung mitochondria. *J. Biol. Chem.* **277**: 26268–26275.

96. Pecqueur, C. *et al.* 2008. Uncoupling protein-2 controls proliferation by promoting fatty acid oxidation and limiting glycolysis-derived pyruvate utilization. *FASEB J.* **22**: 9–18.

97. Bouillaud, F. 2009. UCP2, not a physiologically relevant uncoupler but a glucose sparing switch impacting ROS production and glucose sensing. *Biochim. Biophys. Acta* **1787**: 377–383.

98. Pecqueur, C. *et al.* 2001. Uncoupling protein 2, in vivo distribution, induction upon oxidative stress, and evidence for translational regulation. *J. Biol. Chem.* **276**: 8705–8712.

99. Samudio, I., M. Fiegl & M. Andreeff. 2009. Mitochondrial uncoupling and the Warburg effect: molecular basis for the reprogramming of cancer cell metabolism. *Cancer Res.* **69**: 2163–2166.

100. Ayyasamy, V. *et al.* 2011. Cellular model of Warburg effect identifies tumor promoting function of UCP2 in breast cancer and its suppression by genipin. *PLoS One* **6**: e24792.

Ann. N.Y. Acad. Sci. ISSN 0077-8923

The future: therapy of myocardial protection

David Sanz-Rosa,[1] Jaime García-Prieto,[1] and Borja Ibanez[1,2]

[1]Centro Nacional de Investigaciones Cardiovasculares Carlos III (CNIC), Madrid, Spain. [2]Cardiovascular Institute, Hospital Clínico San Carlos, Madrid, Spain

Address for correspondence: Borja Ibanez, M.D., Ph.D., FESC, Imaging in Experimental Cardiology Laboratory, Atherothrombosis and Imaging Department, Centro Nacional de Investigaciones Cardiovasculares Carlos III (CNIC), c/Melchor Fernández Almagro, 3, Madrid 28029, Spain. bibanez@cnic.es

The main determinant of myocardial necrosis following an acute myocardial infarction (AMI) is duration of ischemia. Infarct size is a strong independent predictor of postinfarction mortality. Interventions able to protect the myocardium from death during an AMI (cardioprotection) are urgently needed. Myocardial injury associated with reperfusion (ischemia/reperfusion injury [I/R]) significantly contributes to the final necrotic size. Duration of ischemia can only be reduced by social and emergency medical services—hospital collaborative programs. However, for a given duration of ischemia, infarct size can be limited by reducing reperfusion injury. Despite the fact that several therapies have been shown to reduce I/R injury in animal models, translation to humans has been frustrating. The cost of developing new drugs able to reduce I/R injury is huge, and this is a major roadblock in the field of cardioprotection. Recent studies have proposed that old, inexpensive drugs—in human use for decades (e.g., β-blockers and cyclosporine, among others)—can reduce I/R injury when administered intravenously before coronary opening. The demonstration of such a cardioprotective effect should have a significant impact in the care of AMI patients.

Keywords: ST elevation myocardial infarction; reperfusion injury; ischemia/reperfusion; infarct size

Introduction

Acute myocardial infarction (AMI) is the result of an acute coronary artery occlusion. Despite that, for a long time, this fact was only inferred from animal studies, the demonstration of coronary artery occlusion in humans with ST-segment elevation AMI (STEMI) was not evident until the work of DeWood *et al.* in the 1980s.[1] Seminal studies performed three decades ago with animal models demonstrated that an early reperfusion (restoration of blood flow into the ischemic myocardium) was able to limit infarct size.[2] A few years later, fibrinolysis was indisputably associated with a reduction in mortality in patients with STEMI.[3] A decade later, primary angioplasty (mechanical reperfusion in the cath lab) was shown to be superior to fibrinolysis.[4] From that point on, primary coronary angioplasty (PCI) has been established as the mainstay treatment for STEMI patients.

When "time is muscle"

The time from the onset of symptoms of AMI (representative of the time of coronary occlusion) and reperfusion (ischemia duration) has been shown to be the strongest determinant of mortality and morbidity in STEMI. In addition, it is known that the duration of coronary occlusion (time from onset of symptoms and reperfusion) is also the major determinant of infarct size. Hence, ischemia shortening is the main therapeutic objective for STEMI patients. Even though reperfusion is the prerequisite for myocardial salvage, the process of restoring blood flow to the ischemic area can induce additional injury to the myocardium—the so-called reperfusion injury,[5] reducing the beneficial effects of reperfusion. In this sense, reperfusion injury can be defined as "the injury caused by the restoration of blood flow after an ischemic episode, leading to death of cells that were only reversibly injured at the time of blood flow

doi: 10.1111/j.1749-6632.2012.06501.x

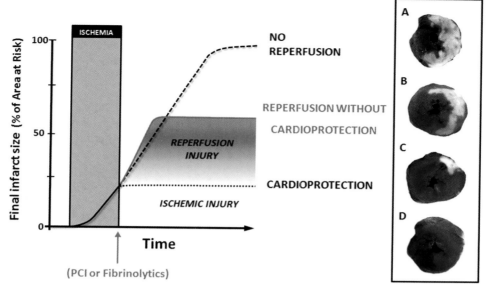

Figure 1. Myocardial death during ischemia and reperfusion. When a coronary artery is occluded, myocardial death grows exponentially. If there is no reperfusion, the final MI size will be the left ventricular area irrigated by the coronary artery (striped line). If the reperfusion occurs in a reasonable time, the MI size is reduced (red line). However, if the reperfusion occurs along with a reduction of reperfusion injury (dotted line), the benefit in MI size is even greater. Pictures on the right show representative mouse hearts after ischemia-reperfusion. TTC staining (red) depicts the viable myocardium, while pale areas are the necrotic myocardium. Pictures have been taken from experiments performed in Ibanez's laboratory (unpublished data).

restoration." The final infarct size is therefore the result of the ischemic and reperfusion damage. For this reason, the term better reflecting this process of myocardial death in a reperfused AMI is myocardial ischemia/reperfusion (I/R) injury. Given that today a vast majority of patients with STEMI are treated with reperfusion, the damage induced in the myocardium is always the result of I/R injury. In clinical practice, the real impact of I/R injury has not been fully determined, as it is also affected by the time of ischemia and other important determinants (i.e., the presence of collaterals, comorbidities, etc.). However, in animal models of myocardial I/R, reperfusion itself can contribute up to 30–40% (Fig. 1).

Strategies shortening the time from STEMI diagnosis to PCI have been widely developed. Beyond social programs that can shorten time from symptom initiation to medical care contact, therapies that can prevent death of endangered myocardium are urgently needed. In this regard, a recent human study[6] was carried out focusing on "system-delay," which is the time from the first contact with the emergency medical service (EMS) to the initiation

of reperfusion therapy in patients with a STEMI. More than 6,000 patients with STEMI undergoing PCI were included in the study and stratified according to system-delay. The authors found that the longer the system-delay the higher the long-term mortality. This study underlines the importance of the cooperation between EMS and hospitals and/or cath labs in order to reduce system-delay.

After recognition of the temporal relationship between coronary occlusion and loss of myocardium, the paradigm, "time is muscle," developed. However, a landmark observation by Reimer's group[7] challenged this paradigm by demonstrating—for the first time in 1986—that the myocardium can be conditioned for future ischemic episodes. In seminal work performed in dog model of AMI, Murry *et al.* observed that brief episodes of ischemia and reperfusion "before" a sustained ischemic insult (i.e., an index episode of AMI) resulted in a significant reduction of final infarct size, compared to dogs in which coronary occlusion was performed straight, despite the same duration of ischemia.[7] They termed this phenomenon "preconditioning." This intervention partially explains why patients with preinfarction angina have better prognosis than patients in which the ischemic episode starts with no prior symptoms.[8] Unfortunately, and for obvious reasons, preconditioning has no role in human STEMI setting. More recently, Vinten-Johansen's group demonstrated (again in a dog model) that brief episodes of coronary occlusion/reperfusion applied after the entire ischemic episode and at the time of reperfusion was also effective in reducing infarct size.[9] They call this intervention "postconditioning." Additional work confirmed activation in the myocardium of the "reperfusion injury salvage kinases" (RISK) group of proteins in both strategies.[10]

Taking the advantage that postconditioning is performed at the time of reperfusion, it has been easily translated into humans with STEMI.[11] The first demonstration that postconditioning was able to reduce myocardial infarct size in humans came from Staat *et al.*,[12] who randomized a selected population of STEMI patients in which stenting was achieved very early after reperfusion to receive either regular reperfusion or brief episodes of coronary occlusion/reperfusion immediately after stenting (with the balloon with which the stent was implanted). They demonstrated that postconditioning reduces enzyme release (a surrogate of infarct size). Following this first report, several attempts have been performed but with discouraging results.[13] The fact that the latter studies obtained negative results and did not replicate the Staat *et al.* study does not necessarily mean that postconditioning does not work. The likely reason for the discrepancy in results is that it is challenging to perform postconditioning in a reasonable time window after reperfusion is achieved. In fact, it has been proposed that the window of cardioprotection for postconditioning is narrow and restricted to the very first minutes after reperfusion. In clinical practice, only a highly selected group of patients would benefit from this strategy, for example, patients with total coronary occlusion that opens with PCI wire progression, low thrombus burden, and in which it is possible to perform direct stenting.

More recently, a new version of myocardial conditioning in STEMI has been reported. Botker *et al.* have reported the first human evidence of remote ischemic (peri)conditioning.[14] "Remote periconditioning" refers to the ability of conditioning the heart during ongoing ischemia by brief periods of ischemia and reperfusion in a remote organ (contrary to pre- and postconditioning, which are performed immediately before or after the index ischemic episode, as was initially described in animal models[15]). More than 300 patients with STEMI were randomized in Botker's trial to receive either remote periconditioning, induced by four cycles of five min of inflation and five min of deflation of a blood-pressure cuff placed in the upper arm, or no conditioning intervention (i.e., regular treatment) during patient transfer to the cath lab, where primary PCI was performed in all patients. This study reported that this easy-to-perform intervention increased myocardial salvage by 33% compared to controls. Future studies should confirm these provocative results.

After the recognition of different forms of conditioning as an effective means to prevent myocardial death during I/R, indentifying the mediators responsible of these phenomena has been of great interest. Among the many drugs that have been used as pharmacological preconditioning mimetics, adenosine has been widely tested in the clinical arena. In the AMISTAD-II trial, more than 2,000 patients presenting with anterior wall AMI were randomized to receive placebo or adenosine for three h, starting within 15 min of reperfusion therapy. As an adjunct to PCI, adenosine showed an 11% reduction in the size of myocardial infarcts, but benefits in terms of clinical outcomes were limited to patients presenting within three hours after the onset of symptoms, and the adenosine dose needed to achieve this effect was high.[16,17] To overcome this dose effect, Desmet *et al.* performed a prospective, single-center, double-blind, placebo-controlled clinical study in which patients with STEMI of less than 12 h were randomized to receive either intracoronary administration of adenosine (4 mg) distal to the occlusion site or matching placebo, immediately before the initial balloon inflation. They found no differences in myocardial salvage index, microvascular obstruction, or crude infarct size, as evaluated by state-of-the-art magnetic resonance imaging (MRI, the gold standard for assessing infarct size in humans).[18] Confirming the MRI results, widely used parameters, such as ST-segment elevation resolution, TIMI perfusion grade, and enzymatic release (among others) were also similar in adenosine-treated patients versus placebo. Finally, authors conclude by detracting

22. Piper, H.M., Y. Abdallah & C. Schafer. 2004. The first minutes of reperfusion: a window of opportunity for cardioprotection. *Cardiovasc. Res.* **61:** 365–371.

23. Griffiths, E.J. & A.P. Halestrap. 1995. Mitochondrial non-specific pores remain closed during cardiac ischaemia, but open upon reperfusion. *Biochem. J.* **307**(Pt 1): 93–98.

24. Oka, N., L. Wang, W. Mi, *et al.* 2008. Cyclosporine a prevents apoptosis-related mitochondrial dysfunction after neonatal cardioplegic arrest. *J. Thoracic Cardiovasc. Surg.* **135:** 123–130, 130 e121–122.

25. Ibanez, B. & J.J. Badimon. 2008. Cyclosporine in acute myocardial infarction. *N. Engl. J. Med.* **359:** 2287; author reply 2288–2289.

26. Piot, C., P. Croisille, P. Staat, *et al.* 2008. Effect of cyclosporine on reperfusion injury in acute myocardial infarction. *N. Engl. J. Med.* **359:** 473–481.

27. Kitakaze, M., M. Asakura, J. Kim, *et al.* 2007. Human atrial natriuretic peptide and nicorandil as adjuncts to reperfusion treatment for acute myocardial infarction (j-wind): two randomised trials. *Lancet* **370:** 1483–1493.

28. Ibanez, B., V. Fuster, J. Jimenez-Borreguero & J.J. Badimon. 2011. Lethal myocardial reperfusion injury: a necessary evil? *Int. J. Cardiol.* **151:** 3–11.

29. Rodriguez-Sinovas, A., Y. Abdallah, H.M. Piper & D. Garcia-Dorado. 2007. Reperfusion injury as a therapeutic challenge in patients with acute myocardial infarction. *Heart Fail. Rev.* **12:** 207–216.

30. Klein, H.H., S. Pich, S. Lindert, *et al.* 1989. Treatment of reperfusion injury with intracoronary calcium channel antagonists and reduced coronary free calcium concentration in regionally ischemic, reperfused porcine hearts. *J. Am. Coll. Cardiol.* **13:** 1395–1401.

31. Gumina, R.J., E. Buerger, C. Eickmeier, *et al.* 1999. Inhibition of the na(+)/h(+) exchanger confers greater cardioprotection against 90 minutes of myocardial ischemia than ischemic preconditioning in dogs. *Circulation* **100:** 2519–2526; discussion 2469–2572.

32. Zeymer, U., H. Suryapranata, J.P. Monassier, *et al.* 2001. The Na(+)/H(+) exchange inhibitor eniporide as an adjunct to early reperfusion therapy for acute myocardial infarction. Results of the evaluation of the safety and cardioprotective effects of eniporide in acute myocardial infarction (escami) trial. *J. Am. Coll. Cardiol.* **38:** 1644–1650.

33. Ishii, H., S. Ichimiya, M. Kanashiro, *et al.* 2005. Impact of a single intravenous administration of nicorandil before reperfusion in patients with st-segment-elevation myocardial infarction. *Circulation* **112:** 1284–1288.

34. Frangogiannis, N.G., C.W. Smith, M.L. Entman. 2002. The inflammatory response in myocardial infarction. *Cardiovasc. Res.* **53:** 31–47.

35. Petzelbauer, P., P.A. Zacharowski, Y. Miyazaki, *et al.* 2005. The fibrin-derived peptide beta15–42 protects the myocardium against ischemia-reperfusion injury. *Nat. Med.* **11:** 298–304.

36. Atar, D., P. Petzelbauer, J. Schwitter, *et al.* 2009. Effect of intravenous fx06 as an adjunct to primary percutaneous coronary intervention for acute st-segment elevation myocardial infarction results of the f.I.R.E. (efficacy of fx06 in the prevention of myocardial reperfusion injury) trial. *J. Am. Coll. Cardiol.* **53:** 720–729.

37. Yellon, D.M. & D.J. Hausenloy. 2007. Myocardial reperfusion injury. *N. Engl. J. Med.* **357:** 1121–1135.

38. Opie, L.H. 2008. Metabolic management of acute myocardial infarction comes to the fore and extends beyond control of hyperglycemia. *Circulation* **117:** 2172–2177.

39. Maroko, P.R., P. Libby, B.E. Sobel, *et al.* 1972. Effect of glucose-insulin-potassium infusion on myocardial infarction following experimental coronary artery occlusion. *Circulation* **45:** 1160–1175.

40. Opie, L.H., K. Bruyneel & P. Owen. 1975. Effects of glucose, insulin and potassium infusion on tissue metabolic changes within first hour of myocardial infarction in the baboon. *Circulation* **52:** 49–57.

41. Fath-Ordoubadi, F. & K.J. Beatt. 1997. Glucose-insulin-potassium therapy for treatment of acute myocardial infarction: an overview of randomized placebo-controlled trials. *Circulation* **96:** 1152–1156.

42. Diaz, R., A. Goyal, S.R. Mehta, *et al.* 2007. Glucose-insulin-potassium therapy in patients with st-segment elevation myocardial infarction. *JAMA* **298:** 2399–2405.

43. Apstein, C.S. & L.H. Opie. 2005. A challenge to the metabolic approach to myocardial ischaemia. *Eur. Heart J.* **26:** 956–959.

44. Nikolaidis, L.A., S. Mankad, G.G. Sokos, *et al.* 2004. Effects of glucagon-like peptide-1 in patients with acute myocardial infarction and left ventricular dysfunction after successful reperfusion. *Circulation* **109:** 962–965.

45. Lonborg, J., N. Vejlstrup, H. Kelbaek, *et al.* 2011. Exenatide reduces reperfusion injury in patients with st-segment elevation myocardial infarction. *Eur. Heart J.* doi: 10.1093/eurheartj/ehr309

46. Freemantle, N., J. Cleland, P. Young, J. Mason & J. Harrison. 1999. Beta blockade after myocardial infarction: systematic review and meta regression analysis. *BMJ* **318:** 1730–1737.

47. Antman, E.M., M. Hand, P.W. Armstrong, *et al.* 2008. 2007 focused update of the acc/aha 2004 guidelines for the management of patients with st-elevation myocardial infarction: a report of the american college of cardiology/american heart association task force on practice guidelines: developed in collaboration with the canadian cardiovascular society endorsed by the american academy of family physicians: 2007 writing group to review new evidence and update the acc/aha 2004 guidelines for the management of patients with st-elevation myocardial infarction, writing on behalf of the 2004 writing committee. *Circulation* **117:** 296–329.

48. Lopez-Sendon, J., K. Swedberg, J. McMurray, *et al.* 2004. Expert consensus document on beta-adrenergic receptor blockers. *Eur. Heart J.* **25:** 1341–1362.

49. Sommers, H.M. & R.B. Jennings. 1972. Ventricular fibrillation and myocardial necrosis after transient ischemia. Effect of treatment with oxygen, procainamide, reserpine, and propranolol. *Arch. Intern. Med.* **129:** 780–789.

50. Ibanez, B., S. Prat-Gonzalez, W.S. Speidl, *et al.* 2007. Early metoprolol administration before coronary reperfusion results in increased myocardial salvage: analysis of ischemic myocardium at risk using cardiac magnetic resonance. *Circulation* **115:** 2909–2916.

51. Ibanez, B., G. Cimmino, S. Prat-Gonzalez, *et al.* 2011. The cardioprotection granted by metoprolol is restricted to its administration prior to coronary reperfusion. *Int. J. Cardiol.* **147:** 428–432.

52. Ibanez, B., V. Fuster, C. Macaya, *et al.* 2011. [Modulation of the beta-adrenergic system during acute myocardial infarction: rationale for a new clinical trial]. *Rev. Esp. Cardiol.* **64**(Suppl 2):28–33.

53. Sanz-Rosa, D., J. García-Prieto, A. Osuna, V. Fuster & B. Ibanez. 2011. β3 adrenergic receptor stimulation protects the heart from ischemia/reperfusion injury. Evolving challenges in promoting cardiovascular health (NYAS meeting, Barcelona).

54. Aragon, J.P., M.E. Condit, S. Bhushan, *et al.* 2011. Beta3-adrenoreceptor stimulation ameliorates myocardial ischemia-reperfusion injury via endothelial nitric oxide synthase and neuronal nitric oxide synthase activation. *J. Am. Coll. Cardiol.* **58:** 2683–2691.

55. Suarez-Barrientos, A., P. Lopez-Romero, D. Vivas, *et al.* 2011. Circadian variations of infarct size in acute myocardial infarction. *Heart* **97:** 970–976.

56. Reiter, R., C. Swingen, L. Moore, T.D. Henry & J.H. Traverse. 2012. Circadian dependence of infarct size and left ventricular function after st elevation myocardial infarction. *Circ Res.* **110:** 105–110.

57. Arroyo Úcar, E., A. Dominguez-Rodriguez, P. Abreu-Gonzalez. 2012. Influence of diurnal variation in the size of acute myocardial infarction. *Med. Intensiva.* **36:** 11–14.

58. Bar, F.W., D. Tzivoni, M.T. Dirksen, *et al.* 2006. Results of the first clinical study of adjunctive CAldaret (MCC-135) in patients undergoing primary percutaneous coronary intervention for ST-Elevation Myocardial Infarction: the randomized multicentre CASTEMI study. *Eur. Heart J.* **27:** 2516–2523.

59. Bates, E., C. Bode, M. Costa, *et al.* 2008. Intracoronary KAI-9803 as an adjunct to primary percutaneous coronary intervention for acute ST-segment elevation myocardial infarction. *Circulation* **117:** 886–896.

60. Lonborg, J., H. Kelbaek, N. Vejlstrup, *et al.* 2010. Cardioprotective effects of ischemic postconditioning in patients treated with primary percutaneous coronary intervention, evaluated by magnetic resonance. *Circ. Cardiovasc. Interv.* **3:** 34–41.

61. Fan, Q., X.C. Yang, Y. Liu, *et al.* 2011. Postconditioning attenuates myocardial injury by reducing nitro-oxidative stress in vivo in rats and in humans. *Clin. Sci. (Lond.)* **120:** 251–261.

62. Garcia, S., T.D. Henry, Y.L. Wang, *et al.* 2011. Long-term follow-up of patients undergoing postconditioning during ST-elevation myocardial infarction. *J. Cardiovasc. Transl. Res.* **4:** 92–98.

Ann. N.Y. Acad. Sci. ISSN 0077-8923

ANNALS OF THE NEW YORK ACADEMY OF SCIENCES

Issue: *Evolving Challenges in Promoting Cardiovascular Health*

The links between complex coronary disease, cerebrovascular disease, and degenerative brain disease

Jason C. Kovacic,[1,2] Jose M. Castellano,[1,2] and Valentin Fuster[1,2,3]

[1]The Zena and Michael A. Wiener Cardiovascular Institute, Mount Sinai School of Medicine, New York, New York.
[2]Marie-Josée and Henry R. Kravis Cardiovascular Health Center, Mount Sinai School of Medicine, New York, New York. [3]The Centro Nacional de Investigaciones Cardiovasculares (CNIC), Madrid, Spain

Address for correspondence: Dr. Valentin Fuster, M.D., Ph.D., Mount Sinai School of Medicine, One Gustave L. Levy Place, Box 1030, New York, NY 10029. valentin.fuster@mountsinai.org

Our appreciation of the complexity of cardiovascular disease is growing rapidly. Consistent with the fact that the vasculature is an omnipresent system that carries blood to every organ in the body, an expanding number of conditions are now known to be directly associated with disturbed cardiovascular function or vascular pathology. In particular, cardiovascular disease has recently been implicated as playing a major role in dementia and other forms of degenerative brain disease. Here, we explore some of the many emerging relationships between cardiovascular risk factors, complex coronary artery disease, cerebrovascular disease, and degenerative brain disease.

Introduction

Gone are the days when cardiovascular disease (CVD) was considered to be just an atherosclerotic plaque accumulation that causes arterial narrowing or occlusion and that may culminate in myocardial infarction or stroke. Today, CVD is understood to be a complex disease process that incites a broad spectrum of maladaptive and pathologic pathways and that may lead to diverse end-organ pathologies, including renal insufficiency, atrial fibrillation, impotence, stroke, and degenerative brain disease (DBD). In this paper, we consider the links between complex coronary artery disease (cCAD), DBD, and cerebrovascular disease.

cCAD

cCAD is a term we have coined that has specific reference to the multisystems nature of advanced atherosclerotic and coronary artery disease.[1] In this regard, the major impact of CVD and cCAD on the physiologic functioning of almost every organ and system in the body is now beginning to be fully appreciated. Along with many other associations, as will be reviewed in this paper, extensive data have also shown a close relationship between cCAD and DBD. In parallel with these widespread biological

associations, a number of seminal clinical studies have recently emerged that, from a different perspective, have reinforced the notion of cCAD. These major clinical studies have had a significant influence on our understanding of cCAD, while at the same time demonstrating that effective treatment of cCAD requires an equally complex therapeutic approach (Table 1). As a result of these studies, sophisticated treatment algorithms have arisen that incorporate elements such as risk stratification, assessment of disease burden, consideration of comorbidities, attention to risk factor modification, optimization of medical therapies, and comprehensive functional assessment of coronary artery disease prior to consideration of revascularization procedures (Table 1). Although the implementation of these clinical algorithms may take time,[2] these data certainly serve the purpose of highlighting the incredible biocomplexity of coronary artery disease and the advanced strategies that are required to make meaningful therapeutic gains.

Complex cerebrovascular disease

Looking beyond the heart, the most obvious initial vascular link to cCAD is that of concomitant carotid artery atherosclerotic disease. We have

Table 1. Recent pivotal clinical trials that have helped to define the nature of complex coronary artery disease

Trial acronym	Major findings	Reference
COURAGE	Optimal medical therapy is an appropriate initial treatment strategy for the majority of patients with stable CAD	Boden *et al.*[47]
BARI-2D	No significant difference in rates of death and major cardiovascular events between diabetic patients with CAD undergoing revascularization and those receiving medical therapy alone	Frye *et al.*[48]
SYNTAX	A series of studies showing that patients with complex coronary anatomy (SYNTAX score ≥ 33) should be triaged to undergo coronary artery bypass surgery rather than PCI	Serruys *et al.*[49–51]
Clinical SYNTAX	The addition of clinical information in the SYNTAX algorithm such as age, and both left ventricular and renal function improves the accuracy of this score for predicting cardiovascular outcomes	Serruys *et al.*[52]
FAME	In patients undergoing PCI, fractional flow reserve (FFR) testing should be used to identify hemodynamically significant coronary lesions prior to stent implantation	Tonino *et al.*[53]
FREEDOM	Ongoing study seeking to define the role of PCI versus bypass surgery in diabetic patients	Fuster *et al.*[54]
PROSPECT	Following an acute coronary syndrome, nonculprit lesions that were responsible for subsequent unanticipated events were frequently angiographically mild, most were thin-cap fibroatheromas or were characterized by a large plaque burden, a small luminal area, or some combination of these characteristics	Stone *et al.*[55]
HRP Bioimage	Ongoing study aiming to discover novel ways to identify patients at risk for near-term CVD events	Muntendam *et al.*[10]

Reproduced and adapted from work by Kovacic and Fuster.[1]

previously noted that a not insignificant number of persons present to medical attention with cCAD and, at the same time, obstructive extracranial carotid artery disease.[3] Recent studies have confirmed that the severity of carotid artery stenosis is significantly correlated to the extent of CAD ($r = 0.255$, $P < 0.001$).[4] Furthermore, the burden of carotid plaque is a strong predictor of future cardiac death and MACE in CAD patients.[5] The revascularization options for obstructive carotid atherosclerosis have been of intense interest and controversy over the last decade, with traditional surgical endarterectomy being compared against the newer modality of percutaneous carotid stenting in numerous studies and registries.[6] Current consensus guideline recommendations place heavy emphasis on whether the patient is symptomatic from their carotid disease and on the severity of the stenosis.[6] While certain scenarios may dictate a specific approach, such as a prior neck procedure with significant scarring favoring stenting rather than endarterectomy,[7] consensus guidelines now suggest a reasonable degree of equipoise in the choice between stenting and endarterectomy (Table 2).[6] The management of concomitant cCAD and carotid disease continues to pose a particular management challenge,[3] with consensus opinion favoring treatment of the most symptomatic territory first.[8]

The carotid arteries have also been the site of intense investigations as to optimal noninvasive imaging modalities for characterizing atherothrombotic disease. Diagnostic advances go hand-in-

36. Kramer, L. *et al.* 1998. Previous episodes of hypoglycemic coma are not associated with permanent cognitive brain dysfunction in IDDM patients on intensive insulin treatment. *Diabetes* **47:** 1909–14.

37. Ho, L. *et al.* 2004. Diet-induced insulin resistance promotes amyloidosis in a transgenic mouse model of Alzheimer's disease. *Faseb J.* **18:** 902–904.

38. Kearney, P.M. *et al.* 2005. Global burden of hypertension: analysis of worldwide data. *Lancet* **365:** 217–223.

39. Novak, V. *et al.* 2010. The relationship between blood pressure and cognitive function. *Nat. Rev. Cardiol.* **7:** 686–698.

40. Hajjar, I. *et al.* 2011. Hypertension, white matter hyperintensities, and concurrent impairments in mobility, cognition, and mood: the Cardiovascular Health Study. *Circulation* **123:** 858–65.

41. White, W.B. *et al.* 2011. Average daily blood pressure, not office blood pressure, is associated with progression of cerebrovascular disease and cognitive decline in older people. *Circulation* **124:** 2312–2319.

42. Kovacic, J.C. *et al.* 2011. Cellular senescence, vascular disease, and aging: part 1 of a 2-part review. *Circulation* **123:** 1650–1660.

43. Donmez, G. *et al.* 2010. SIRT1 suppresses beta-amyloid production by activating the alpha-secretase gene ADAM10. *Cell* **142:** 320–332.

44. Kim, D. *et al.* 2007. SIRT1 deacetylase protects against neurodegeneration in models for Alzheimer's disease and amyotrophic lateral sclerosis. *Embo. J.* **26:** 3169–79.

45. Huang, T.C. *et al.* 2011. Resveratrol protects rats from abeta-induced neurotoxicity by the reduction of iNOS expression and lipid peroxidation. *PLoS One* **6:** e29102.

46. Launer, L.J. *et al.* 2010. Lowering midlife levels of systolic blood pressure as a public health strategy to reduce late-life dementia: perspective from the Honolulu Heart Program/Honolulu Asia Aging Study. *Hypertension* **55:** 1352–1359.

47. Boden, W.E. *et al.* 2007. Optimal medical therapy with or without PCI for stable coronary disease. *N. Engl. J. Med.* **356:** 1503–1516.

48. Frye, R.L. *et al.* 2009. A randomized trial of therapies for type 2 diabetes and coronary artery disease. *N. Engl. J. Med.* **360:** 2503–2515.

49. Serruys, P.W. *et al.* 2009. Percutaneous coronary intervention versus coronary-artery bypass grafting for severe coronary artery disease. *N. Engl. J. Med.* **360:** 961–972.

50. Serruys, P.W. *et al.* 2009. Assessment of the SYNTAX score in the SYNTAX study. *EuroIntervention* **5:** 50–56.

51. Sianos, G. *et al.* 2005. The SYNTAX score: an angiographic tool grading the complexity of coronary artery disease. *EuroIntervention* **1:** 219–227.

52. Garg, S. *et al.* 2010. A new tool for the risk stratification of patients with complex coronary artery disease: the Clinical SYNTAX score. *Circ. Cardiovasc. Interv.* **3:** 317–326.

53. Tonino, P.A. *et al.* 2009. Fractional flow reserve versus angiography for guiding percutaneous coronary intervention. *N. Engl. J. Med.* **360:** 213–224.

54. Farkouh, M.E. *et al.* 2008. Design of the Future REvascularization Evaluation in patients with Diabetes mellitus: Optimal management of Multivessel disease (FREEDOM) Trial. *Am. Heart J.* **155:** 215–223.

55. Stone, G.W. *et al.* 2011. A prospective natural-history study of coronary atherosclerosis. *N. Engl. J. Med.* **364:** 226–35.

Ann. N.Y. Acad. Sci. ISSN 0077-8923

ANNALS OF THE NEW YORK ACADEMY OF SCIENCES

Issue: *Evolving Challenges in Promoting Cardiovascular Health*

Optimal lipid targets for the new era of cardiovascular prevention

Vimal Ramjee,[1] Danny J. Eapen,[2] and Laurence S. Sperling[2]

[1]J. Willis Hurst Internal Medicine Residency, Emory University School of Medicine, Atlanta, Georgia. [2]Department of Medicine, Section of Preventive Cardiology, Emory University, Atlanta, Georgia.

Address for correspondence: Laurence Sperling, 1365 Clifton Road NE, Building A, Suite 2200, Atlanta, GA 30322. lsperli@emory.edu

Optimal lipid targets (OLT) should be the goal for all individuals treated in the new era of cardiovascular (CV) disease prevention. Evidence supports that average LDL cholesterol (LDL-C) values in Westernized populations are not optimal. Lessons from nature and science support a physiologic LDL-C target of <70 mg/dL. Clinical trial evidence further supports optimal LDL-C targets, although several critical questions remain unanswered. Using a calculated LDL-C may have limitations in clinical practice. Non-HDL-C cholesterol may be a better predictor of outcomes, and should therefore be provided on all laboratory reports. Specific HDL cholesterol (HDL-C) targets are significantly more complicated. Although a low HDL-C predicts a less favorable outcome independent of LDL-C level, an HDL-C level > 50 mg/dL is associated with lower CV risk. Clinical trials on HDL-C have thus far been disappointing. OLT should be the goal for all individuals as an important part of addressing global CV risk.

Keywords: optimal lipid; OLT; cardiovascular; HDL; LDL; triglyceride

Background

With a growing cardiometabolic phenotype in the United States and globalization of the Westernized lifestyle, the prevalence of cardiovascular risk factors continues to increase at a rapid rate.[1–4] Risk factors, including tobacco use, dyslipidemia, diabetes, and hypertension, among others, contribute to the pathogenesis of atherosclerotic vascular disease. As such, the prevention of cardiovascular disease (CVD) takes a multifaceted approach directed toward the optimal treatment of each of these distinct factors.

Physiology and nature

In contrast to other risk factors, low-density lipoprotein cholesterol (LDL-C) has been established as the major necessary and sufficient factor for the development and progression of atherosclerosis.[5] The relevance of optimal lipid targets as they pertain to the prevention of CVD is grounded in the central role that lipids play in the initiation and development of atherothrombotic lesions. Oxidative modification of LDL-C exists within a spectrum, from minimally modified (mmLDL) to significantly oxidized (oxLDL), the latter of which is believed to initiate the process of atherogenesis by binding to scavenger receptors on macrophages and smooth muscle cells.[5,6] An imbalance between lipid burden and physiologic capacity can result in an overwhelmed protective-immunologic response, giving rise to death of foam cells and destabilization of the lipid-rich core, with subsequent increased risk of plaque rupture, thrombosis, and fatal events.

Although increased longevity of our species may unmask disease entities that otherwise may not have been described in our ancestors, atherosclerosis has been defined as a process primarily related to the lipid burden that our culture and diet has brought forth, and not our longevity. Anthropological observations, for instance, show little to no evidence of atherosclerosis among preagricultural and twentieth-century hunter-gatherers in the seventh and eighth decades of life.[7,8] In addition, the absence of atherosclerosis has been demonstrated

doi: 10.1111/j.1749-6632.2012.06478.x

across virtually all mammalian species from a spectrum of ages.[9,10]

It is likely that the low prevalence of CVD in hunter-gatherers was partially attributable to a higher level of physical activity, but also because they did not possess LDL-C levels overwhelming the physiologic capacity of the body. The LDL-C level of hunter-gatherers, neonates, wild primates, and wild mammals has been extrapolated to a range of approximately 30–70 mg/dL in several studies.[8,11–14] Compared to our predecessors, the average American adult today has an LDL-C level of 130 mg/dL (or at least two- to fourfold more than hunter-gatherers), a 50% chance of establishing atherosclerosis by the age of 50 years, and self-reports of being relatively physically inactive ($\sim$60–65% of the U.S. population).[1,15–17] Some believe that the discordance between the Paleolithic genome and our modern day diet, with the rapid advent of processed, refined, and fat-laden products, accounts at least in part for the current endemic of CVD.[11] Others, however, argue that dietary indiscretion, independent of genetic consideration, is accountable for the current state of CVD.[17] Being that modern day humans are the only animals with an LDL-C >80 mg/dL, it is not surprising that we have the highest prevalence of atherosclerotic CVD.[11] Taken together, these findings underscore the notion that atherosclerosis is not a natural part of our physiology or of aging, but a chronic, smoldering inflammatory process that is a result of extrinsic sociocultural factors. Furthermore, these data support the concept that a lower LDL-C of less than 70 mg/dL corresponds to our physiologic level and is therefore optimal in ensuring a lifetime free of cardiovascular events.

Science and trials

Although current NCEP ATP III guidelines recommend therapeutic targeting of LDL-C to less than 70 mg/dL only in the highest-risk individuals (Table 1), emerging data continue to support the need for further reduction of LDL-C in other populations.[18–22]

O'Keefe *et al.*[11] completed multiple univariate regression analyses in which crucial points of disease and event progression relating to LDL-C were defined on the basis of several large RCTs.[23–32] In their analysis, the point limitation of atherosclerotic progression corresponded to an LDL-C of 67 mg/dL, and the coronary heart disease (CHD) event rate approached 0% at an LDL-C of 57 mg/dL and

Table 1. Current NCEP guidelines for LDL-C and non-HDL-C

Risk category	LDL-C goal (mg/dL)	Non-HDL-C goal (mg/dL)
Highest risk (CHD, CHD equivalent, or 10-year risk score >20%)	<100 (<70[a])	<130 (<100[a])
Moderately high risk (≥2 minor risk factors, or 10-year risk score 10–20%)	<130 (<100[b])	<160 (<130[b])
Moderate risk (≥2 risk factors, or 10-year risk score < 10%)	<130	<160
Low risk (<2 risk factors, or 10-year risk score <10%)	<160	<190

[a]Optional goal for highest-risk patients.
[b]Optional goal for higher-risk patients.
Data from Refs. 18 and 22.

30 mg/dL in primary and secondary prevention, respectively.[11]

Several large randomized controlled trials (RCTs) have demonstrated findings consistent with this analysis in the setting of both primary and secondary prevention.[28–31,33–36] In the West of Scotland Coronary Primary Prevention Study, for instance, 6,595 men (age, 45–64 years) were randomized to receive either 40 mg pravastatin or placebo over a mean of 4.9 years.[30] There were clinically significant event reductions in the pravastatin group for nonfatal myocardial infarction (RRR 31%, $P < 0.001$), any coronary event (RRR 31%, $P < 0.001$), and death from all cardiovascular causes (RRR 32%, $P = 0.033$).[30] In the Air Force/Texas Coronary Atherosclerosis Prevention Study (AFCAPS/TexCAPS), 6,605 men and women (age, 45–73 years) were randomized to lovastatin (20–40 mg) or placebo and followed over an average of 5.2 years.[28] Compared with placebo, the treatment group showed significant reductions in first acute major coronary events (RR: 0.63; 95% CI: 0.50–0.79; $P < 0.001$), myocardial infarction (RR: 0.60; 95% CI: 0.43–0.83; $P = 0.002$), unstable angina (RR: 0.68; 95% CI: 0.49–0.95; $P = 0.02$), coronary revascularization procedures (RR: 0.67; 95% CI: 0.52–0.85; $P = 0.001$), coronary events

Table 2. Lower is better: intensive versus conservative statin therapy in patients with ACS

Trial	N	Intervention arms	Baseline LDL (mg/dL)	LDL difference at 1 year (mg/dL)	Events (% per year)	
					Statin/more	Control/less
PROVE IT-TIMI 22	4162	A80, P40	101.3	25.1	11.3	13.1
IDEAL	8888	A40/80, S20/40	102.1	21.3	5.2	6.3
TNT	10001	A80, A10	97.4	24	4	5.4
A to Z	4497	S40/80, P/S20	80.8	11.6	3.6	3.8
SEARCH	12064	S80, S20	96.7	15.1	7.2	8.1

Note: Data from Refs. 31, 33–36.

(RR: 0.75; 95% CI: 0.61–0.92; $P = 0.006$), and cardiovascular events (RR: 0.75; 95% CI: 0.62–0.91; $P = 0.003$).[28] In the Anglo-Scandinavian Cardiac Outcomes Trial-Lipid Lowering Arm (ASCOT-LLA),[29] 10,305 participants (age, 40–79 years) were randomized to receive either atorvastatin 10 mg or placebo over an average of 5 years. The study was stopped after a median of 3.3 years given a clinically significant reduction in total cardiovascular events (RR: 0.79; 95% CI: 0.69–0.90; $P = 0.0005$), and total coronary events (RR: 0.71; 95% CI: 0.59–0.86; $P = 0.0005$) in the treatment arm.[29] Collectively, these trials, among others, provide clear evidence that lowering of LDL-C in the primary prevention population results in significant cardiovascular event reduction.

In addition, recent large secondary prevention trials have demonstrated the benefits of further reduction of LDL-C with intensive statin therapy compared to standard dose treatment (Table 2). In the PROVE IT-TIMI 22 trial, for instance, 4,162 postacute coronary syndrome patients (mean age, 58 years) were randomized to high-dose atorvastatin versus standard-dose pravastatin and followed for an average of two years.[31] The primary endpoint was defined as a composite of death from any cause, myocardial infarction, documented unstable angina requiring rehospitalization, revascularization with either percutaneous coronary intervention or coronary-artery bypass grafting (if these procedures were performed at least 30 days after randomization), and stroke. There was a significant reduction of the primary endpoint in the atorvastatin group (median LDL-C, 62 mg/dL) compared with the pravastatin group (median LDL-C, 95 mg/dL; RR: 0.16; 95% CI: 0.05 to 0.26; $P = 0.005$).[31] In the IDEAL study, 8,888 secondary prevention patients (mean age, 62 years) were randomized to high-dose atorvastatin versus usual-dose simvastatin with a 5-year follow-up.[36] In this study, there was a significant reduction of coronary events (Hazard ratio (HR): 0.84; 95% CI: 0.76–0.91; $P < 0.001$) and nonfatal MI (HR: 0.83; 95% CI: 0.71–0.98; $P = 0.02$) in the atorvastatin group (mean LDL-C, 81 mg/dL) compared with the simvastatin group (mean LDL-C, 104 mg/dL). In the TNT study, 10,001 secondary prevention patients (age, 35–75 years) were randomized to low- or high-dose atorvastatin and were followed for five years.[35] The high-dose arm (mean LDL-C, 77 mg/dL) demonstrated a significant reduction of any coronary event (HR: 0.79; 95% CI: 0.73–0.86; $P < 0.001$), and any cardiovascular event (HR: 0.81; 95% CI: 0.75–0.87; $P < 0.001$) compared with the low-dose arm (mean LDL-C, 101 mg/dL).[35]

In the second-cycle of the Cholesterol Treatment Trialists' meta-analysis, Baigent *et al.*[20] collectively assessed 39,612 secondary prevention subjects (weighted mean baseline LDL-C, 97.7 mg/dL) from five RCTs of more intensive versus less intensive statin therapy (Table 2). The weighted mean difference in LDL-C at one year was 19.7 mg/dL, with significantly fewer major coronary events in the more intensive statin group compared to the less intensive statin group (RR: 0.74; 95% CI: 0.65–0.85; $P < 0.0001$). More remarkably, in the combined analysis of all 26 RCTs, which included both primary and secondary prevention individuals, there was a 22% reduction in major vascular events for every 38.6 mg/dL (1 mmol/L) decrease in LDL-C regardless of initial LDL-C level. Of note, there was a linear relationship between LDL-C reduction and relative risk reduction (RRR) of major vascular events. With a fixed RRR independent of starting LDL-C level, benefit may be further extrapolated to a 40% CV event reduction for every 2 mmol/L decrease in

Ann. N.Y. Acad. Sci. ISSN 0077-8923

ANNALS OF THE NEW YORK ACADEMY OF SCIENCES
Issue: *Evolving Challenges in Promoting Cardiovascular Health*

Controversies in blood pressure goal guidelines and masked hypertension

Robert A. Phillips

University of Massachusetts Medical School, Worcester, Massachusetts

Address for correspondence: Robert A. Phillips, M.D., Ph.D., 55 Lake Avenue North, AC4-242, Worcester, MA 01655. Robert.Phillips@umassmemorial.org

In uncomplicated hypertension, <140/90 mmHg is the treatment goal for individuals aged 18–79 and between 140 mmHg and 150 mmHg in those 80 years of age. Inhibitors of the renin–angiotensin–aldosterone system, as well as calcium channel blockers, are universally accepted as first-line therapy in uncomplicated hypertension, but controversy exists over the role of thiazide diuretics and beta blockers. Because at similar blood pressure (BP) levels, African Americans have more target organ damage than whites, a lower goal of <135/85 mmHg is recommended. In patients with coronary artery disease, diabetes, and chronic kidney disease, <130/80 mmHg is recommended. Masked hypertension, defined as normal clinic BP with a high average self-monitored or ambulatory BP, is prevalent in those with chronic kidney disease, diabetes, and obstructive sleep apnea. Masked hypertension is associated with worse outcome. Ambulatory BP monitoring for those at risk for masked hypertension needs to be incorporated into guidelines.

Keywords: blood pressure; guidelines; masked hypertension; essential hypertension

Introduction

Over the past decade, multiple guidelines and consensus statements on the treatment of essential hypertension (HTN) have been issued from the United States, the United Kingdom, Japan, Europe, Canada, and international organizations.[1–7] The focus of this review is to critically assess blood pressure (BP) goal guidelines and explore controversies in uncomplicated essential HTN in the elderly, African Americans, diabetics, chronic kidney disease (CKD), and coronary artery disease (CAD). In addition, first-line antihypertensive therapy, combination therapy, and the emerging problem of masked hypertension will be briefly reviewed.

Uncomplicated hypertension

There is universal agreement that BP should be <140/90 mmHg in patients <80 years of age.[1–7] However, the basis for this position in patients age ≥65 with isolated systolic hypertension is scant, as no trial has achieved an average systolic BP <143 mmHg. Those individuals who achieved an SBP <140 mmHg in these trials may not have had incremental benefit. For example, in the Systolic Hypertension in the Elderly Program (SHEP), where the entry criteria was a systolic BP (SBP) >170 mmHg, those who achieved an SBP <160 mmHg had a 33% reduction in stroke, and a further 5% reduction was accrued in those with SBP <150 mmHg.[8] However, there was no further benefit seen in those who achieved an SBP <140 mmHg. Nevertheless, all guidelines have an SBP goal of <140 mmHg in those aged <80.

In those aged ≥80, guidance is available from the Hypertension in the Very Elderly Trial (HYVET).[9] The study hypothesis was that in patients age ≥80 with SBP between 160 and 199 mmHg, antihypertensive therapy with a BP goal of <150/80 mmHg would be efficacious. The primary endpoint of the trial was any stroke (fatal or nonfatal), excluding TIAs. Secondary endpoints included death from any cause, death from cardiovascular causes, death from cardiac causes, and death from stroke.

HYVET randomized a total of 3,845 patients from Europe, China, Australia, and Tunisia to either

doi: 10.1111/j.1749-6632.2012.06489.x

indapamide 1.5 mg sustained release (SR) or placebo. At each visit (or at the discretion of the investigator), if needed to reach the target BP (SBP <150 mmHg and DBP <80 mmHg), perindopril 2 mg or 4 mg or matching placebo could be added. At two years, 25.8% of patients in the active treatment group were receiving indapamide alone, 23.9% were receiving indapamide and perindopril 2 mg, and 49.5% were receiving indapamide and perindopril 4 mg. At two years, mean standing BP levels had decreased by 13.6/7.0 mmHg in the placebo group (demonstrating once again the power of placebo), and by 28.3/12.4 mmHg in the active treatment group, where the SBP was on average 143 mmHg.

At the two-year follow-up, compared to placebo, antihypertensive drug therapy with indapamide, plus perindopril if needed, reduced all-cause mortality by 21%. This is the first major hypertension trial to show a reduction in mortality. In addition, fatal or nonfatal stroke was reduced by 30%, fatal stroke by 39%, cardiovascular death by 23%, and heart failure by 64%.

HYVET results have been incorporated into two guidelines. Basing their recommendation on the SBP goal in HYVET, the U.K. NICE guidelines recommend a BP <150 mmHg,[2] whereas the American College of Cardiology (ACC)/American Heart Association (AHA) recommend a more aggressive target SBP goal of 140–145 mmHg.[4]

Initiation of antihypertensive therapy in uncomplicated HTN: Where is the debate?

In uncomplicated hypertension, all guidelines recommend either an angiotensin-converting enzyme inhibitor (ACEI), an angiotensin receptor blocker (ARB), or a calcium channel blocker (CCB) as first-line therapy (Table 1).[1-7] Virtually all guidelines, with the exception of UK NICE,[2] also recommend diuretic as a potential first-line therapy. Because of concerns of metabolic disturbances associated with thiazide diuretics (particularly hyperglycemia), in the absence of heart failure, NICE relegate thiazides to second-line therapy for patients of African descent, and third line in other ethnic groups. NICE recommends addition of sprionolactone as fourth-line therapy.

Recommendations regarding β blockers are mixed, as some guideline committees are more concerned than others about their relative ineffectiveness compared to other agents in stroke prevention

Table 1. Recommendations for initiation of antihypertensive therapy according to guidelines/consensus statements issued from national and international organizations

Country/region	ACEI/ARB/ CCB	Diuretic	β blocker
USA-JNC 7[1]	Yes	Yes	Yes
Europe[6]	Yes	Yes	Yes
Japan[5]	Yes	Yes	Yes/no
Canada[7]	Yes	Yes	Yes/no
USA – ACC[4]	Yes	Yes	No
International (Blacks)[3]	Yes	Yes	No
UK[2]	Yes	No	No

ACEI, angiotensin-converting enzyme inhibitor; ARB, angiotensin receptor blocker; CCB, calcium channel blocker.

in the elderly, and the concern about their potential to exacerbate diabetes. After review of the data, and recognizing the pharmacological and possible clinical heterogeneity of β blockers, the European Society of Hypertension recommended continued use of β blockers as first-line therapy.[6] The Japanese Society of Hypertension and the Canadian Hypertension Education Program recommend β blockers in young patients, but recommends other drugs in the elderly or in those with glucose intolerance or diabetes.[5,7] The NICE guidelines have relegated β blockers to fourth-line therapy, except in young patients with "an intolerance or contraindication to ACE inhibitors and angiotensin II antagonists or women of child-bearing potential or people with evidence of increased sympathetic drive."[2]

Combination therapy

While the choice of initial therapy is important, since most patients require at least two drugs for BP control (JNC 7), more emphasis needs to be placed on determining the most efficacious drug combination. Combining drugs with different mechanisms of actions is a physiological approach associated with more effective BP lowering (Fig. 1).[5] The most effective combinations include an ACEI or an ARB combined with a CCB or thiazide diuretic, or a β blocker combined with a CCB. Because of the increased incidence of diabetes, the combination of β blocker and thiazide diuretic is not recommended

disease (PVD) or diabetes mellitus plus one or more additional cardiovascular risk factors, but without left ventricular dysfunction.

In 75% of participants, ramipril was dosed at night, and therefore this study can be considered a nocturnal BP treatment trial. ABP measurements were taken in a subgroup of 38 patients from the HOPE study with PVD, defined as a history of intermittent claudication and an ankle-to-brachial systolic pressure index of <0.9 by Doppler ultrasonography at rest. ABP measurements were taken for 24 h at baseline before study randomization and then after one year of randomized treatment.

Twenty-four-hour ABP was significantly reduced in the ramipril group compared with the placebo group (12/5 mmHg vs. 2/1 mmHg, $P = 0.03$). A marked reduction in BP was observed in the ramipril group at night (16/7 mmHg, $P < 0.001$). Daytime ABP measurements also showed a reduction in BP in the ramipril group compared with the placebo group; however, the between-group comparison was not significant.[33] The reduced nocturnal BP most likely influenced the outcome of the trial.

In the overall trial, ramipril reduced the occurrence of the primary endpoint, MI, stroke, or death from cardiovascular causes (14% vs. 17.8%, relative risk [RR] 0.78, $P < 0.001$). Among secondary outcomes, ramipril versus placebo reduced the rate of death from any cause (10.4% vs. 12.2%, RR 0.84, $P = 0.005$), death from cardiovascular causes (6.1% vs. 8.1%, RR 0.74, $P < 0.001$), complications related to diabetes (6.4% vs. 7.6%, RR 0.84, $P = 0.03$), hospitalization for heart failure (3.0% vs. 3.4%, RR 0.88, $P = 0.25$), and revascularization procedures (16% vs. 18.3%, RR 0.85, $P = 0.002$). Ramipril also significantly reduced the occurrence of MI, heart failure, and stroke versus placebo (all $P <$ 0.001).

Conflicts of interest

The author declares no conflicts of interest.

References

1. Chobanian, A.V., G.L. Bakris, H.R. Black, et al. 2003. The seventh report of the Joint National Committee on Prevention, Detection, Evaluation, and Treatment of High Blood Pressure: the JNC 7 Report. JAMA **289:** 2560–2571.
2. National Institute for Health and Clinical Excellence (NICE). Clinical management of primary hypertension in adults. Clinical guideline #127. 2011. http://www.nice.org.uk/guidance/CG127
3. Flack, J.M., D.A. Sica, G. Bakris, et al. 2010. Management of high blood pressure in blacks. Hypertension **56:** 780–800.
4. Aronow, W.S., J.L. Fleg, C.J. Pepine, et al. 2011. ACCF/AHA 2011 expert consensus document on hypertension in the elderly: a report of the American College of Cardiology Foundation Task Force on Clinical Expert Consensus Documents Developed in collaboration with the American Academy of Neurology, American Geriatrics Society, American Society for Preventive Cardiology, American Society of Hypertension, American Society of Nephrology, Association of Black Cardiologists, and European Society of Hypertension. J. Am. Coll. Cardiol. **57:** 2037–2114.
5. Ogihara, T., K. Kikuchi, H. Matsouka, et al. 2009. The Japanese Society of Hypertension Guidelines for the Management of Hypertension (JSH 2009). Hypertens. Res. **32:** 3–1007.
6. Mancia, G., S. Laurent, E. Agabiti-Rosei, et al. 2009. Reappraisal of European guidelines on hypertension management: a European Society of Hypertension Task Force document. Blood Pressure **18:** 308–347.
7. Rabi, D.M., S.S. Daskalopoulou, R.S. Padwal, et al. 2011. The 2011 Canadian Hypertension Education Program recommendations for the management of hypertension: blood pressure measurement, diagnosis, assessment of risk, and therapy. Can. J. Cardiol. **27:** 415–433.
8. Perry, H.M.J., B.R. Davis, T.R. Price, et al. 2000. Effect of treating isolated systolic hypertension on the risk of developing various types and subtypes of stroke: the Systolic Hypertension in the Elderly Program (SHEP). JAMA **284:** 465–471.
9. Beckett, N.S., R. Peters, A.E. Fletcher, et al. 2008. Treatment of hypertension in patients 80 years of age or older. N. Engl. J. Med. **358:** 1887–1898.
10. Jamerson, K., M.A. Weber, G.L. Bakris, et al. 2008. Benazepril plus amlodipine or hydrochlorothiazide for hypertension in high-risk patients. N. Engl. J. Med. **359:** 2417–2428.
11. Jamerson, K.A., R. Devereux, G.L. Bakris, et al. 2011. Efficacy and duration of benazepril plus amlodipine or hydrochlorthiazide on 24-hour ambulatory systolic blood pressure control. Hypertension **57:** 174–179.
12. Ernst, M.E., B.L. Carter & J.N. Basile. 2009. All Thiazide-like diuretics are not chlorthalidone: putting the ACCOMPLISH study into perspective. J. Clin. Hypertens. **11:** 5–10.
13. Klag, M.J., P.K. Whelton, B.L. Randall, et al. 1997. End-stage renal disease in African-American and white men. 16-year MRFIT findings. JAMA **277:** 1293–1298.
14. Appel, L.J., J.T. Wright, T. Greene, et al. 2010. Intensive blood-pressure control in hypertensive chronic kidney disease. N. Engl. J. Med. **363:** 918–929.
15. Schrier, R.W., R.O. Estacio, A. Esler, et al. 2002. Effects of aggressive blood pressure control in normotensive type 2 diabetic patients on albuminuria, retinopathy and strokes. Kidney Int. **61:** 1086–1097.
16. Estacio, R.O., B.F. Jeffers, N. Gifford, et al. 2004. Effect of blood pressure control on diabetic microvascular complications in patients with hypertension and type 2 diabetes. Diabetes Care B54–B64.
17. The ACCORD Study Group. 2010. Effects of intensive blood-pressure control in type 2 diabetes mellitus. N. Engl. J. Med. **362:** 1575–1585.

18. Brown, W.W. & W.F. Keane. 2001. Proteinuria and cardio-vascular disease. *Am. J. Kid. Dis.* **38:** S8–S13.

19. Upadhyay, A., A. Earley, S.M. Haynes, *et al.* 2011. Systematic review: blood pressure target in chronic kidney disease and proteinuria as an effect modifier. *Ann. Intern. Med.* **154:** 541–548.

20. Nissen, S.E., E.M. Tuzcu, P. Libby, *et al.* 2004. Effect of antihypertensive agents on cardiovascular events in pateints with coronary disease and normal blood pressure. *JAMA* **292:** 2217–2226.

21. Sipahi, I., E.M. Tuzcu, P. Schoenhagen, *et al.* 2006. Effects of normal, pre-hypertensive, and hypertensive blood pressure levels on progression of coronary atherosclerosis. *J. Am. Coll. Cardiol.* **48:** 833–838.

22. Rosendorff, C., H.R. Black, C.P. Cannon, *et al.* 2007. Treatment of hypertension in the prevention and management of ischemic heart disease: a scientific statement from the American Heart Association Council for High Blood Pressure Research and the Councils on Clinical Cardiology and Epidemiology and Prevention. *Circulation* **115:** 2761–2788.

23. Messerli, F.H., G. Mancia, C.R. Conti, *et al.* 2006. Dogma disputed: can aggressively lowering blood pressure in hypertensive patients with coronary artery disease be dangerous? *Ann. Intern. Med.* **144:** 884–893.

24. Fagard, R.H., J.A. Staessen, L. Thijs, *et al.* 2007. On-treatment diastolic blood pressure and prognosis in systolic hypertension. *Arch. Intern. Med.* **167:** 1884–1891.

25. Haller, H., S. Ito, J.L. Izzo, *et al.* 2011. Olmesartan for the delay or prevention of microalbuminuria in type 2 diabetes. *N. Engl. J. Med.* **364:** 907–917.

26. Pickering, T.G., K. Davidson, W. Gerin, *et al.* 2002. Masked hypertension. [Editorial]. *Hypertension* **40:** 795–796.

27. Mann, S.J., G.D. James, R.S. Wang, *et al.* 1991. Elevation of ambulatory systolic blood pressure in hypertensive smokers: a case-control study. *JAMA* **265:** 2226–2228.

28. Ben-Dov, I.Z., D. Ben-Ishay, J. Mekler, *et al.* 2007. Increased prevalence of masked blood pressure elevations in treated diabetic subjects. *Arch. Intern. Med.* **167:** 2139–2142.

29. Pogue, V., M. Rahman, M. Lipkowitz, *et al.* 2009. Disparate estimates of hypertension control from ambulatory and clinic blood pressure measurements in hypertensive kidney disease. *Hypertension* **53:** 20–27.

30. Baguet, J.P., P. Levy, G. Barone-Rochette, *et al.* 2008. Masked hypertension in obstructive sleep apnea syndrome. *J. Hypertens.* **26:** 885–892.

31. Bobrie, G., G. Chatellier, N. Genes, *et al.* 2004. Cardiovascular prognosis of "masked hypertension" detected by blood pressure self-measurement in elderly treated hypertensive patients. *JAMA* **291:** 1342–1349.

32. Yusuf, S., P. Sleight, J. Pogue, *et al.* 2000. Effects of an angiotensin-converting-enzyme inhibitor, ramipril, on cardiovascular events in high-risk patients. The Heart Outcomes Prevention Evaluation Study Investigators [see comments]. *N. Engl. J. Med.* **342:** 145–153.

33. Svensson, P., U. de Faire, P. Sleight, *et al.* 2001. Comparative effects of ramipril on ambulatory and office blood pressures. *Hypertension* **38:** e28–e32.

34. Giles, T.D. & G.E. Sander. 2001. Beyond the usual strategies for blood pressure reduction: therapeutic considerations and combination therapies. *J. Clin. Hypertens.* **3:** 346–353.

Ann. N.Y. Acad. Sci. ISSN 0077-8923

Evolving diagnostic and prognostic imaging of the various cardiomyopathies

Javier Sanz[1,2]

[1]The Zena and Michael A. Wiener Cardiovascular Institute, [2]Marie-Josée and Henry R. Kravis Center for Cardiovascular Health, Mount Sinai School of Medicine, New York, New York

Address for correspondence: Javier Sanz, Cardiovascular Institute, Mount Sinai Hospital, One Gustave L Levy Place, Box 1030, New York, NY 10029. Javier.Sanz@mssm.edu

Several noninvasive imaging modalities, particularly cardiac magnetic resonance (CMR), have of late provided important diagnostic and prognostic insights into various cardiomyopathies. Myocardial delayed enhancement on CMR after administration of contrast accurately delineates a scar, a powerful marker of poor prognosis in dilated cardiomyopathy. Also in heart failure, loss of integrity of the cardiac sympathetic nervous system, as demonstrated by reduced myocardial uptake of the radioisotope meta-iodo-benzylguanidine with nuclear imaging similarly provides information on outcomes. The presence/absence of a scar on CMR has emerged as an important diagnostic and/or prognostic tool for specific cardiomyopathies, such as Tako-Tsubo, sarcoidosis, or hypertrophic cardiomyopathy. In addition, the quantification of the myocardial parameter $T2^*$ on CMR has been validated for accurate quantification of iron myocardial overload and as the strongest predictor for incident heart failure. In these diseases, coronary angiography with computed tomography (CT) may be very useful in ruling out underlying coronary disease noninvasively.

Keywords: cardiomyopathy; imaging; magnetic resonance; computed tomography; nuclear medicine

Introduction

The evaluation of the patient with myocardial disease relies heavily on the use of imaging modalities. Morphologic and functional parameters, such as left ventricular (LV) volumes, mass, and ejection fraction, are time-honored indices of cardiac performance and patient outcome that are employed daily in routine clinical practice for decision making. In this regard, transthoracic echocardiography (TTE) remains the mainstay of myocardial imaging due to its widespread availability, low cost, and ability to provide concomitant information on valvular function, atrial size, and, semiquantitatively, right ventricular size and contractility. In addition, stress imaging with either TTE or nuclear modalities is extensively used to noninvasively detect the presence of coronary artery disease, the most common underlying etiology of dilated cardiomyopathy (DCM).

During the last decade, there have been substantial advances in the field of myocardial imaging,

including TTE, nuclear techniques, computed tomography (CT), and, particularly, cardiac magnetic resonance (CMR). Beyond the traditional evaluation of ventricular volume/function and the presence of ischemia and viability, novel approaches enable detection of myocardial metabolism, scarring, edema, microvascular obstruction, hemorrhage, or neuronal integrity. This review summarizes recent developments in the field of myocardial imaging.

Ischemic cardiomyopathy

One of the main determinants of clinical management of patients with ischemic cardiomyopathy has traditionally been the presence or absence of significant viability, which can be detected with several of the aforementioned imaging modalities. This is because previous retrospective studies showed strong associations between viability presence and improved survival if surgical revascularization was performed.[1] However, a prospective study published

doi: 10.1111/j.1749-6632.2012.06490.x
Ann. N.Y. Acad. Sci. 1254 (2012) 123–130 © 2012 New York Academy of Sciences.

in 2011 challenged this notion. A substudy of the Surgical Treatment for Ischemic Heart Failure trial evaluated the influence of viability on outcomes of patients with ischemic cardiomyopathy randomized to intensive medical therapy with or without surgical revascularization. Approximately 50% of participants ($n = 601$) underwent viability imaging with single photon emission CT (SPECT) and/or dobutamine TTE. After five years, all-cause death (the primary endpoint) occurred in 37% of patients with significant viability in comparison with 51% of those without ($P = 0.003$). However, after adjustment for clinical covariates such as age, renal function, LV volumes, LV ejection fraction, and others, the presence of viability was not an independent predictor of survival. Importantly, there was no influence of type of therapy on the main outcome, although patients with viability who received surgery experienced significant reductions in a secondary endpoint of combined death and cardiovascular hospitalization.[2]

Regarding the evaluation of ischemic cardiomyopathy with CMR, a number of parameters have been identified in the last few years that offer prognostic value. Myocardial infarct can be depicted as bright areas in the myocardium with the use of postcontrast delayed enhancement (DE) imaging that demonstrates myocardial scarring or necrosis as bright regions (Fig. 1). Moreover, further characterization of the infarct by defining areas of dense scarring (higher signal) versus those with intermixed fibrosis and viable myocytes (border zone or "gray" zone due to its intermediate signal intensity) has shown promise in the identification of arrhythmic substrates[3] and of patients with higher risk of future events.[4] These reports highlight one of the evolving applications of myocardial imaging: the guidance of device implantation. Scar characterization with DE CMR may provide information additive to that of LVEF in determining potential benefit of automatic implantable cardiac defibrillators.[5] The presence and location of a scar may be also useful to predict response (or lack of thereof) to cardiac resynchronization therapy. A recent study of TTE and speckle tracking employed a threshold of <16.5% radial strain to determine the presence of a scar as validated with CMR DE. Besides the presence of substantial dyssynchrony and optimal placement of the LV pacing lead at the site of latest mechanical activation, both predictors of improved outcomes, the

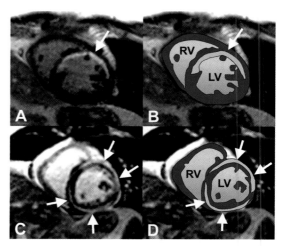

Figure 1. Examples of delayed myocardial enhancement (bright signal) using CMR. Panels A and C correspond to the original short-axis images of the heart. In panels B and D, the myocardium (red), cardiac cavity (pink), and the area of delayed enhancement (yellow) are highlighted. The patient in panels A and B has an anterior myocardial infarction (arrows) involving approximately 50% of the transmural thickness of the wall. Panels C and D represent a patient with myocarditis, where the enhancement is circumferential and predominantly subepicardial and intramyocardial (arrows), indicating nonischemic etiology. LV, left ventricle; RV, right ventricle.

presence of a transmural scar at the pacing site was independently associated with higher rates of death and heart failure hospitalization.[6] In the patient after an acute myocardial infarction, the presence of microvascular obstruction and/or intramyocardial hemorrhage by CMR has also been associated with impaired outcomes.[7,8]

Nonischemic cardiomyopathies

When facing the patient with newly diagnosed DCM, the first question is commonly one of whether the underlying etiology is coronary disease. Invasive coronary angiography is then performed in many centers; however, noninvasive imaging approaches may provide a reasonable alternative. In this regard, CT angiography has shown high accuracy in ruling out significant coronary artery disease in DCM of unknown etiology.[9] The rationale for using CMR DE as an alternative is that most patients with ischemic DCM will have scars in an ischemic pattern (predominantly subendocardial in a vascular territory), while patients with nonischemic DCM will have either no scar or nonischemic patterns (predominantly intramyocardial or subepicardial without a clear vascular distribution, Fig. 1).[10] A recent study performed in the United Kingdom reported cost-effectiveness of CMR with combined DE and coronary imaging versus invasive angiography in this context, although these results may not apply to environments with different CMR or catheterization costs.[11]

Various recent studies have evaluated the prognostic value of DE in cardiomyopathy. In a retrospective single-center investigation of 857 patients with both ischemic and nonischemic etiologies, the presence of myocardial DE predicted outcomes beyond LVEF and adjusting for multiple covariates. After a median follow-up of 4.4 years, survival free from transplantation was 87% in those with normal LVEF and no DE, and 60% in those with both LV dysfunction and myocardial scar. Interestingly, survival was comparable (approximately 77%) in patients with LV dysfunction and no scar versus patients with DE and normal LVEF, suggesting that the presence of a scar may be as powerful a prognosticator as LVEF.[12] These findings were more recently confirmed in a multicenter study involving 1,560 patients.[13] Not only the presence but the amount of scar is associated with impaired outcomes after accounting for LVEF.[14] Moreover, in a cohort of 103 patients with implantable defibrillators indicated for primary prevention, no appropriate therapies occurred in those with nonischemic DCM and absent myocardial DE over a median follow-up period of approximately 1.5 years,[15] again suggesting a potential role of imaging in selection of candidates for device therapy. Longer follow-up will be needed to determine the practical significance of these findings. Despite these promising results, the visualization of a scar with CMR is limited by the fact that the presence of normal reference myocardium is necessary for DE imaging. Novel approaches are exploring the possibility of also detecting and quantifying diffuse myocardial fibrosis,[16] an exciting application that may open new ways of evaluating myocardial disease.

Another interesting approach that has been revisited for risk stratification in patients with ischemic and nonischemic DCM is the visualization of myocardial sympathetic activity with [123I]meta-iodobenzylguanidine (MIBG) SPECT. MIBG is a norepinephrine analogue that accumulates in the presynaptic neuronal terminals, allowing detection

with a gamma-camera. A recent multicenter trial, including 961 patients with severe LV dysfunction, evaluated the use of the ratio of myocardial to mediastinal uptake in planar imaging for the prediction of events. Those with reduced myocardial uptake (ratio < 1.6), indicative of loss of neuronal integrity, had a 37% two-year rate of heart failure progression, life threatening arrhythmias or cardiac death in comparison with 15% in those with preserved uptake ($P < 0.001$).[17]

Left ventricular noncompaction

Noncompaction cardiomyopathy is an incompletely understood disease resulting from interruption of normal myocardial development and leading to the persistence of a prominently trabeculated inner myocardial layer. The natural history of this disease is largely unknown, but it may present as DCM.[18] Uncertainties extend to the appropriate criteria for diagnosis, which is commonly based on different TTE findings.[19] A novel approach based on the ratio of noncompacted (trabeculated) to compacted myocardium by CMR was recently proposed. In comparison with controls and patients with DCM or hypertrophic cardiomyopathy (HCM), a ratio >20% correctly identified 94% of patients with presumed noncompaction.[20] These preliminary results will require further validation. Similarly, LV noncompaction may be accompanied by prominent fibrosis as demonstrated by DE,[21] but the implications of this finding remain to be elucidated.

Cardiac sarcoidosis

Cardiac involvement is clinically evident in only a minority of patients with sarcoidosis, usually in the form of DCM and/or arrhythmias. Nevertheless, cardiac sarcoid is a main cause of death, and both autopsy and, more recently, advanced imaging studies reveal myocardial lesions in a substantial proportion of cases.[22] Two imaging modalities have an important role in the evaluation of cardiac sarcoidosis, CMR and positron emission tomography (PET). CMR is the technique with probably highest specificity, and can detect the presence of myocardial edema (likely reflecting active inflammation) as well as focal areas of scarring, commonly in basal segments. In a recent series of 81 patients with biopsy-proven extracardiac sarcoid, the presence of DE identified cardiac involvement in 26% of patients, in comparison with 12% by standard clinical criteria. In addition, there was a trend for higher incidence of cardiac death or symptomatic arrhythmia in those patients with DE, although events were too few to reach statistical significance.[23] PET, probably the most sensitive modality, can detect areas of inflammatory activity, as reflected by increased uptake of [18F]fluorodeoxyglucose (FDG), with or without regionally decreased perfusion. Recently, the coefficient of variation in myocardial FDG accumulation, defined as standard deviation divided by average uptake, has been proposed as a more specific quantitative parameter to determine cardiac sarcoid involvement and to follow the effects of corticosteroid therapy.[24]

Acute myocarditis and related disorders

A number of cardiac disorders may present clinically as chest pain with positive troponin and normal coronary arteries on invasive angiography. CMR may be useful in the differential diagnosis, particularly if combined with endomyocardial biopsy as both tests appear to be complementary.[25] The most common underlying disease in these patients is acute myocarditis.[26] The value of CMR in myocarditis evaluation relies on the combination of detection of wall motion abnormalities on cine imaging, myocardial edema with T2-weighted sequences, early diffuse myocardial postcontrast enhancement on T1-weighted imaging, and DE.[27] Some of the abnormalities in the acute phase, such as myocardial edema, may resolve and be absent in the chronic phase, where the patient may present with DCM. In these cases, DE is typically located in the intramyocardial and/or subepicardial layers and may persist but retrospective diagnosis may be difficult. It has recently been suggested that CMR should

be performed within the first two weeks after the acute episode in order to maximize the probability of reaching the correct diagnosis.[28] Another entity that may resemble an acute coronary syndrome but with angiographically normal coronary arteries is stress-induced or Takotsubo cardiomyopathy. Believed to be secondary to catecholamine toxicity on the myocytes, the typical form of Takotsubo presents with acute apical wall motion abnormalities (apical "ballooning") that resolve over time. According to a recent prospective multicenter CMR study,[29] enrolling 256 patients with Takotsubo cardiomyopathy, this form can be seen in over 80% of the cases, with the remainder demonstrating atypical patterns. Of these, concomitant right ventricular involvement may be associated with slower recovery. Myocardial edema and early postcontrast enhancement can be noted in the majority of the patients, whereas <10% (typically those with higher troponin levels) will demonstrate mild, patchy DE.[29] In the appropriate clinical scenario, CT coronary angiography may also be useful to rule out coronary disease in patients with clinical presentation resembling an acute coronary syndrome (Fig. 2).

Iron overload cardiomyopathy

Abnormal iron deposition can occur in hereditary hemochromatosis or in different conditions, particularly if they require multiple blood transfusions. In these diseases, cardiac involvement is a leading cause of mortality.[30] The deposition of iron in the myocardium leads to disturbance of the tissue magnetic properties that can be detected in a completely noninvasive fashion with CMR. On appropriate imaging sequences, the presence of iron

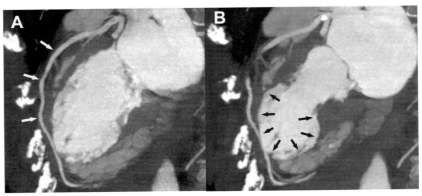

Figure 2. Mid-diastolic (panel A) and end-systolic (panel B) frames of a cardiac CT in a patient with acute chest pain and features suggestive of Takotsubo's cardiomyopathy. Mid-diastole demonstrates a widely patent left anterior descending coronary artery (white arrows), whereas the apical ballooning typical of this disease is noted in end-systole (black arrows).

Ann. N.Y. Acad. Sci. ISSN 0077-8923

ANNALS OF THE NEW YORK ACADEMY OF SCIENCES

Issue: *Evolving Challenges in Promoting Cardiovascular Health*

The evolving landscape of quality measurement for heart failure

Ashley A. Fitzgerald,[1,2] Larry A. Allen,[1,2] and Frederick A. Masoudi[1,2]

[1]Division of Cardiology, Department of Medicine, University of Colorado Anschutz Medical Campus, Aurora, Colorado.
[2]Colorado Cardiovascular Outcomes Research (CCOR) Consortium, Colorado

Address for correspondence: Frederick A. Masoudi, M.D., M.S.P.H., University of Colorado Anschutz Medical Campus, Mailstop B132, 12401 E. 17th Avenue, Aurora, CO 80045. Fred.Masoudi@ucdenver.edu

Heart failure (HF) is a major cause of mortality and morbidity, representing a leading cause of death and hospitalization among U.S. Medicare beneficiaries. Advances in science have generated effective interventions to reduce adverse outcomes in HF, particularly in patients with reduced left ventricular ejection fraction. Unfortunately, effective therapies for heart failure are often not utilized in an effective, safe, timely, equitable, patient-centered, and efficient manner. Further, the risk of adverse outcomes for HF remains high. The last decades have witnessed the growth of efforts to measure and improve the care and outcomes of patients with HF. This paper will review the evolution of quality measurement for HF, including a brief history of quality measurement in medicine; the measures that have been employed to characterize quality in heart failure; how the measures are obtained; how measures are employed; and present and future challenges surrounding quality measurement in heart failure.

Keywords: quality measurement; heart failure; outcomes

Introduction

The goal of health care is to help people live longer and better lives. Therefore, the extent to which health care delivery accomplishes this overall goal represents the quality of that care. The Institute of Medicine's (IOM) report, *Crossing the Quality Chasm: A New Health System for the 21st Century*, defines quality as "the degree to which health care systems, services, and supplies for individuals and populations increase the likelihood for desired health outcomes in a manner consistent with current professional knowledge."[1] The IOM further defined six domains of the highest quality health care: effectiveness—providing services based on scientific knowledge to all who could benefit and refraining from providing services to those not likely to benefit; safety—avoiding harm to patients from the care that is intended to help them; patient-centeredness—providing care that is respectful of and responsive to individual patient preferences, needs, and values and ensuring that patient values guide all clinical decisions; timeliness—reducing waits and sometimes harmful delays for both those who receive and those who give care; efficiency—avoiding waste, including waste of equipment, supplies, ideas, and energy; and equity—providing care that does not vary in quality because of personal characteristics such as gender, ethnicity, geographic location, and socioeconomic status.

Poor quality results from errors in any one of the characteristics of high-quality health care: unsafe practices; use of ineffective therapies; application of the wrong therapy to the wrong patient; delayed delivery of care; use of resource intensive care for marginal benefit; and differential health care delivery strictly based on age, gender, race or ethnicity. Deficits in the quality of health care are also framed as deriving from three types: underuse (i.e., the failure to provide a beneficial therapy); overuse (i.e., the provision of a therapy without significant benefit or for which the risks outweigh the possible advantages); or misuse (i.e., medical errors or other sources of potentially avoidable complications).[2]

Ultimately, the quality of care cannot be understood without accurate measurement. While the

doi: 10.1111/j.1749-6632.2012.06483.x

concept of quality is seemingly intuitive, developing a rigorous quantitative underpinning of quality assessment has proven more challenging. As with other areas of science in medicine, quality measurement has evolved as the result of a body of knowledge resulting from a rigorous study as described below.

Certain conditions are more amenable to quality measurement than others. Heart failure has been a particular focus of quality measurement efforts for several reasons. First, heart failure has a high prevalence—affecting an estimated 5.7–6.6 million adults in the United States. Second, it has an important effect on individual and population health. Heart failure is the most common cause of hospital admission in the older U.S. population.[3] Elderly Medicare patients hospitalized for heart failure have a higher readmission rate within 30 days—more than 26%—than for any other medical condition.[4] Patients with the syndrome are also at high risk for other adverse consequences, including death and poor quality of life.[5,6] As a corollary, because of its prevalence and poor outcomes, the financial consequences of heart failure are substantial—projected to account for more than $44 billion in direct costs in the United States in 2015, or almost one in $12 that will be spent on cardiovascular diseases.[7] Finally, the evidence base for treating heart failure is extensive, resulting in robust practice guidelines that provide the basis for the development of some of the measures that are used to characterize quality.[8]

A historical perspective of quality measurement

Quality measurement, seemingly a recent development in medicine, is not a new concept. In the early 20th century, the surgeon Ernest Amory Codman (Fig. 1) first proposed the measurement of surgical outcomes when he left his traditional surgical practice to found the "End Results Hospital" in Boston, which routinely described and reported the quality of the care it delivered.[9] However, like many visionary ideas, Codman's systematic approach to quality measurement would not be embraced for decades.

The prevailing model of quality assessment in health care over most of the 20th century diverged from Codman's vision of universal quality measurement, consisting largely of committees focusing on medical care and utilization review. In 1983,

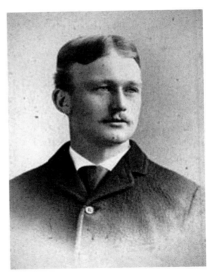

Figure 1. Ernest Amory Codman (source, http://commons.wikimedia.org/).

the Medicare Utilization and Quality Control Peer Review Organization Program was founded with the responsibility of identifying "outliers:" hospitals or practitioners whose care fell well outside the spectrum of normal.[10] These approaches reflected a philosophy that suboptimal quality was rare, sporadic, and the responsibility of only a few individual providers or institutions.

Ultimately, it was recognized that failures to achieve optimal quality in medical care were endemic and resulted primarily from systematic failures to deliver the best care.[10] Efforts to measure medical quality reflected this philosophical shift. In 1992, the Health Care Financing Administration (HCFA, now the Centers for Medicare and Medicaid Services, or CMS) implemented a national effort to measure the quality of care of Medicare patients with acute myocardial infarction (AMI): the Cooperative Cardiovascular Project (CCP).[11] The CCP focused on evidence-based processes of care for AMI (e.g., aspirin, beta blockers, and thrombolytic agents). In an observational follow-up study in four participating states, CCP investigators found that between 1992 and 1995 performance on key process quality indicators improved significantly with associated declines in mortality.[12] Contemporaneously, a substantial effort was dedicated to understanding the quality of care for cardiovascular surgery.[13,14]

A systematic understanding of the quality of care for heart failure developed more slowly. Based upon the perceived success of the CCP and local measurement projects dedicated to heart failure,[15] the CMS launched the National Heart Failure Project (NHF) in 1999 as part of a broader effort to understand and improve the quality of care for health conditions of greatest importance to Medicare beneficiaries. The NHF Project focused upon four inpatient processes of care: assessment of left ventricular ejection fraction; the use of angiotensin-converting enzyme inhibitors in patients with left ventricular systolic dysfunction; providing complete heart failure discharge instructions; and providing smoking cessation counseling in current or recent smokers. Baseline measurements of the four process measures were conducted in 1998–1999 before quality improvement efforts by state Quality Improvement Organizations and repeated subsequently in 2000–2001. The measurements for this project identified significant and widespread gaps in the quality of heart failure care at the beginning of the last decade.[16,17] Subsequently, the CMS and The Joint Commission (TJC) harmonized their measures of inpatient care. Hospitals were first required to submit these performance metrics for the CMS reimbursement ("pay-for-reporting") and for TJC accreditation.[18]

Since the inception of the NHF Project, the landscape of quality measurement for heart failure has evolved dramatically. The scope of measurement has expanded beyond processes of care, the uses of measurement have expanded beyond reporting and accreditation alone, and the opportunities for collecting data have grown. These changes and the associated challenges will be addressed below.

What is measured?

The conceptual framework proposed by Avedis Donabedian in 1966 underlies most contemporary efforts to assess quality of care for medical conditions, including heart failure.[19] Donabedian described three distinct dimensions of quality: structures, processes, and outcomes of care. These dimensions are interrelated, in that high-quality structures should result in a higher likelihood of providing appropriate processes of care, which in turn should result in better patient outcomes.

Structural measures

Structures of care characterize the health care environment, such as personnel, facilities, training, certification, and the implementation of protocols. Perhaps the most commonly employed structural measures are case volume for procedures. Structural measures are convenient because they are often easy to measure; however, they are most often employed when other types of measures are not feasible because of typically weak relationships between structures of care and health outcomes. In the area of heart failure, structural measures have generally not been employed, in large part because more robust process and outcomes measures for heart failure are available. It is worth mentioning that a volume–outcome relationship in heart failure care exists; in a study of Medicare beneficiaries in 4,679 U.S. hospitals, larger volume hospitals had modestly but significantly lower 30-day risk-standardized mortality.[20] However, there is substantial overlap in the mortality distribution among the strata of heart failure case volume, suggesting that this structural characteristic discriminates poorly despite the statistical significance of the relationship.

Process measures

Process measures characterize the care that is delivered to patients. Examples include the prescription of medications, the performance of procedures, and the provision of education. Processes of care measures are calculated by identifying patients with an indication for a particular therapy in the absence of any contraindication (denominator) and assess the proportion that receives the therapy (numerator). Strong evidence is a prerequisite for process measures, which generally focus on those aspects of care that are unequivocally recommended (i.e., class I or III recommendations in clinical practice guidelines). However, while necessary, evidence alone is not sufficient. Process measures must also be interpretable, actionable, valid, reliable, and feasible to calculate.[21,22] Thus, only a subset of evidence-based processes of care qualify for consideration as quality measures. Furthermore, while a larger group of measures may be suitable for the purposes of feedback, benchmarking, and quality improvement, only a subset are considered adequately robust for the purposes of accountability (i.e., public reporting or pay-for-performance), as discussed below.[23]

Table 1. ACC/AHA/PCPI performance measures

Measure	Care setting	Attribution
LVEF assessment	Inpatient	Facility
	Outpatient	Practitioner
ACE (or ARB) for LVSD	Inpatient	Facility
	Outpatient	Practitioner
Beta blocker for LVSD	Inpatient	Facility
	Outpatient	Practitioner
Postdischarge appointment	Inpatient	Facility
Symptom assessment	Outpatient	Practitioner
Symptom management*	Outpatient	Practitioner
Patient self-care education*	Outpatient	Practitioner
ICD counseling*	Outpatient	Practitioner

*Measures proposed for quality improvement purposes but not for accountability.
Adapted from Ref. 24

Several process measures exist to characterize heart failure care. As mentioned above, the CMS, in conjunction with TJC, have used the four "core" heart failure measures in their hospital quality program. More recently, the American College of Cardiology (ACC) and American Heart Association (AHA), in conjunction with the Physician Consortium for Performance Improvement (PCPI), developed a broader group of process measures to assess both inpatient and outpatient care (Table 1).[24]

Process measures have important strengths. First, because they are invariably based upon the most robust evidence; they possess strong face validity.[21] Further, when properly constructed, process measures do not require risk adjustment, further lending credibility and interpretability.[25] However, such measures are also limited for several reasons, including the following: they apply only to those patients who qualify for the measure denominator;[26] they assess only a small fraction of the processes of care that are routinely delivered; and performance on many process measures, particularly those that are components of accountability programs, has reached very high levels, such that process measures for which performance is "topped out" fail to discriminate among institutions.[27] Further complicating their practical use, accurate determination of denominator exclusions can pose additional challenges; in particular, retrospective determination of contraindications to therapy is often problematic for many heart failure therapies.[27] Also notably, the

process measures that are currently widely used to characterize heart failure quality focus entirely on eliminating underuse; issues of overuse and misuse are not addressed.

Finally, the relationship between quality of care as determined by process performance measures and important patient outcomes has been controversial. In a study from the OPTIMIZE registry, an analysis comparing patients who received processes of care with those who did not found that only beta-blocker therapy—which is not currently used by the CMS/TJC as part of the hospital quality measurement program—and ACE inhibitor therapy were associated with better patient outcomes.[28] A subsequent analysis from the same registry focusing on hospital-level performance found that the relationship between these processes and outcomes were substantially attenuated and only beta-blocker prescription was modestly associated with lower mortality.[29] In a third study using the same registry, hospital-level performance, measured by established quality measures as well as others that have not been widely used, found modest associations with quality- and hospital-level outcomes.[30] The seemingly discrepant results of these studies may be in part explained by a number of factors, including differences in the level of analysis (patient vs. institution level), differences in the time frame of follow-up for outcomes, and the fact that performance on established measures was generally higher with less variation than for other measures. However, other studies have found that the relationship between process measures used to characterize the quality of care for heart failure and patient outcomes is weak,[31] raising questions about the extent to which existing process measures as adequate reflections of quality of care.

Outcome measures

Because of the limitations of the process of care measures in heart failure, there has been an increasing focus on directly measuring heart failure outcomes. With respect to patients with heart failure, widely used outcomes measures include mortality and readmission following hospitalization.[32,33] These outcomes are appealing on a clinical and policy level because they occur relatively frequently in patients who have been hospitalized with heart failure. Readmission is also associated with significant costs.[34] At least among patients for whom administrative data are available (e.g., Medicare fee-for-service patients), these outcomes are relatively easy to collect longitudinally.

The ACC and AHA have developed standards for outcome measures, which include (1) a clearly defined patient sample; (2) clinically coherent variables for risk adjustment; (3) high-quality and timely data; (4) specification of a reference time before which risk adjustment variables are collected and after which outcomes are ascertained; (5) a standardized period of assessment for outcomes (e.g., one month or one year rather than in-hospital); (6) an analytic approach that accounts for clustering of patients within systems; and (7) transparency of the methods used.[35]

The primary strength of outcome measures is that they are patient centered and meaningful not only to individual patients, but also to society as a whole.[25,36] Further, unlike process measures, outcome measures do not require restriction to patients who qualify for a specific therapy. Finally, outcome measures reflect the overall performance of health systems. There are several important limitations that have to be considered with outcome measures, including (1) risk adjustment techniques must be fair in order to account for differences in case mix; (2) decisions about when to measure the outcome of interest are arbitrary; (3) some meaningful outcomes (e.g., health status) are difficult to measure in large populations and across health systems; (4) some meaningful outcomes are relatively rare, limiting power to differentiate important variations in institutional performance; and (5) attributing the outcome to the condition of interest can be complicated by coexisting conditions.[36]

Furthermore, there is a need for caution in interpreting individual outcomes in the context of potentially competing outcomes. This phenomenon is particularly important in patients with heart failure. In a study in the United States of almost seven million Medicare beneficiaries hospitalized for heart failure between 1993 and 2006, there were dramatic declines in the mean length of hospital stay (8.81–6.33 days), in-hospital mortality (8.5–4.3%), and 30-day mortality (12.8–10.7%).[37] However, discharges to skilled nursing facilities simultaneously increased from 13.0% to 19.9%. Further, 30-day readmission rates increased from 17.2% to 20.1%. The assessment of multiple patient outcomes in this study demonstrates the importance of attempting to represent the overall patient experience through simultaneous capture of potential competing outcomes.

Composite measures

Composite measures have been constructed and deployed to address the proliferation of numerous measures of care quality and the need to ensure that these measures comprehensively represent health care quality.[38] Indeed, a substantial challenge of interpretation of various measures within different domains of quality is the lack of association between different metrics within hospitals.[39] Composite measures allow for data reduction to simplify presentation and interpretation and promote better integration of multiple metrics into a more comprehensive assessment of provider performance. However, these advantages come at a cost: standard psychometric properties of composites can be more complex to determine, methods for scoring (e.g., all-or-none vs. any vs. weighting) can lead to different conclusions, and problems with missing data can be amplified.[38] Currently, there are no widely used composite measures to characterize heart failure care, which creates challenges in interpreting the collective importance of individual quality metrics.

How is it measured?

Ultimately, the value of any quality measure depends fundamentally upon the integrity of the data that serves as its foundation. Measuring quality requires commitment, planning, and resources. Contemporary quality measurement relies upon data obtained from administrative sources (i.e., data collected by payers for the purposes of billing), clinical chart abstraction, or clinical registries. Each of these approaches has strengths and limitations.

Administrative data (also known as claims data) from payers typically include large numbers of patients systematically and are relatively inexpensive to use. However, because administrative data are generated primarily to facilitate billing, they often do not provide adequate clinical detail or may be discordant with clinical reality. Further, they are often not generated in a timely manner and are limited only to those patients who are covered by the health plan or system from which they are derived.

In contrast, chart abstraction provides substantially greater clinical detail, thus lending greater face validity to the data. However, chart abstraction is labor intensive and relies entirely on available documentation, which is not standardized and may be incomplete. Clinical data from chart abstraction are used to calculate the process performance measures for heart failure that are reported on the CMS Hospital Compare website.

Clinical registries—observational databases of a clinical condition, procedure, therapy, or population—are perhaps the most effective approach to measuring quality.[40] In the area of heart failure, the AHA Get With The Guidelines Heart Failure (GWTG-HF) program is perhaps the best-known example with a national scope. Unlike administrative data, registries provide clinically granular data. In contrast to data from chart abstraction, registries apply data quality processes and implement standard definitions.[41] Registries thus ensure that critical data elements are consistently collected, and that they are defined identically across care settings. Further, linkages with supplemental data sources such as claims data can provide the benefits of both clinical and administrative data. Such clinical–longitudinal databases create the opportunity to study process–outcome associations. However, because registries are often voluntary, they can be limited by selection bias. Other considerations with clinical registries are the barriers to creating such databases include the administrative burden of current privacy regulations, the difficulty of integrating data collection more seamlessly into clinical care, and the scarcity of funding to support and create current and future registries.

A number of clinical registries have been developed to characterize the quality of inpatient heart failure care.[42–45] These registries have played an important role in shaping quality improvement efforts in heart failure and have the potential to inform future clinical trials, guidelines, and health policy for heart failure.[40]

The proliferation of electronic health records (EHR) promises to enhance further the value of clinical registries and quality measurement. EHRs have the potential to combine and the automated systematic capture of administrative databases with the detailed clinical data of prospective registries chart reviews. However, this potential is not guaranteed; without data standards across EHR platforms, the promise of ubiquitous electronic data sources will not be recognized. Existing registries can help guide

what data are critical to capture within EHR, provide feedback on care and patient outcomes based on data obtained from EHRs, and integrate data collection into clinical care.[40]

How are measurements used?

Quality measurements for heart failure are employed on both on a local and national level. Locally, quality measurements serve to provide feedback to physicians and both inpatient and outpatient care facilities, with how they are performing based on national standards, and overall adherence to the national guidelines and performance measures. Registries such as the AHA GWTG-HF Registry provide users with periodic feedback on performance with respect to processes of care.[44]

However, the use of measures of quality in heart failure has expanded well beyond the important areas of feedback, benchmarking, and quality improvement. As part of its hospital quality program, the CMS made hospital-level data available online for the public beginning in 2005. Performance data—both for processes of heart failure care, 30-day risk-adjusted mortality after heart failure hospitalization, and 30-day risk-adjusted readmission after heart failure readmission—are accessible at the CMS Hospital Compare website.[46] The CMS has also incorporated heart failure quality as part of its "value-based purchasing" program with the hopes of stimulating higher quality care through the use of financial incentives.[47] Although the CMS pay-for-quality programs focus on a wide range of medical conditions, heart failure remains a focus because of its impact on the health of Medicare beneficiaries.

Future challenges

There remains a critical need for further evolution in the quality measurement in heart failure. Generally, quality measurement for heart failure has focused principally on the inpatient setting. This has been the case largely for practical reasons; reliable access to outpatient data has been limited. However, much of the care for heart failure is delivered in the outpatient setting. The prospects for measuring the quality of outpatient care are improved with the development of outpatient cardiovascular registries and the increased penetrance of EHRs.[44,48] However, these registry programs still face the challenge of standardizing data collection across a wide range of practices and clinical data collection platforms.

Furthermore, quality measurement for heart failure has generally focused on underuse and has largely ignored issues around the costs of care or safety. Given the unsustainable trajectory of health care expenditures in the United States, future quality efforts can no longer turn a blind eye to costs. Thus, rather than focusing simply upon the underuse of care, quality measurement must also consider overuse and the value of therapies (defined as the outcomes of healthcare as a function of the cost of delivering that care).[49,50] The measurement of heart failure readmissions—which are undesirable for the patient and invariably incur costs for society—represents an indirect initial foray into characterizing the value of heart failure care. Processes of care that are particularly expensive, such as implantable cardioverter defibrillators, represent specific targets for measures of value, especially as there is evidence of both underuse and overuse of ICD therapy.[51,52] The ACC/AHA have described explicit methodology for measuring value and efficiency; however, important challenges in operationalizing such measurements persist.[53]

Overuse or misuse can create threats to patient safety. For example, in the case of heart failure, aldosterone antagonists reduce the risk of death and hospitalization in carefully selected patients,[54] but risk causing hyperkalemia, particularly in patients with poor renal function. Unfortunately, these agents are often prescribed to patients who are not good candidates for therapy because of renal insufficiency,[55] which has been linked to higher rates of hospitalization for hyperkalemia.[56] Measurement of misuse, while itself also challenging, could ensure that the full potential of therapies that are useful for some but impart higher risk for others, are deployed in a manner that maximizes the population benefit of these therapies.

Other arenas for improvement in quality measurement include (1) leveraging proliferating information technology to improve data sources and provide real-time feedback on quality; (2) constructing process measures with stronger relationships to important health outcomes; (3) the use of patient-centered outcomes such as physical function, symptoms, and quality of life as metrics of quality; (4) focusing on patient subgroups that are underrepresented in clinical trials, such as the el-

derly;[57] (5) reducing disparities in care and outcomes for racial and ethnic minorities;[58,59] and (6) expanding measurement into the realms of palliative and end-of-life care, which are often relevant to many patients with heart failure.[60]

Conclusions

The measurement of quality of care for heart failure has evolved and expanded substantially over the last decade. The focus of measurement, the methods whereby measurement is performed, and the uses of measurement will continue to change in the coming years. Although the future may be unclear, it is certain that quality measurement is intrinsic to delivering medical care for heart failure patients. To this extent, Ernest Codman's vision of understanding and reporting health care quality has been realized.

Conflicts of interest

The authors declare no conflicts of interest.

References

1. Committee on Quality of Health Care in America, I. o. M. 2001. Crossing the Quality Chasm: A New Health System for the 21st Century. National Academy Press. Washington, DC.
2. Agency for Healthcare Research and Quality. 2002. Improving Health Care Quality. Rockville, MD. http://www.ahrq.gov/news/qualfact.htm. Accessed 26 Dec 2011.
3. DeFrances, C.J. *et al.* 2008. 2006 National Hospital Discharge Survey. National Health Statistics. Division of Health Care Statistics, Centers for Disease Control and Prevention, National Center for Health Statistics, Hyattsville, MD. http://www.ncbi.nlm.nih.gov/pubmed/18841653. Accessed 26 Dec 2011.
4. Jencks, S.F., M.V. Williams & E.A. Coleman. 2009. Rehospitalizations among patients in the Medicare fee-for-service program. *N. Engl. J. Med.* **360:** 1418–1428.
5. Masoudi, F.A., E.P. Havranek & H.M. Krumholz. 2002. The burden of chronic congestive heart failure in older persons: magnitude and implications for policy and research. *Heart Failure Rev.* **7:** 9–16.
6. Allen, L.A. *et al.* 2011. Identifying patients hospitalized with heart failure at risk for unfavorable future quality of life. *Circ. Cardiovasc. Qual. Outcomes* **4:** 389–398.
7. Heidenreich, P.A. *et al.* 2011. Forecasting the future of cardiovascular disease in the United States: a policy statement from the American Heart Association. *Circulation* **123:** 933–944.
8. Hunt, S.A. *et al.* 2005. ACC/AHA 2005 guideline update for the diagnosis and management of chronic heart failure in the adult-summary article: a Report of the American College of Cardiology/American Heart Association Task Force on Practice Guidelines (Writing Committee to Update the 2001

Guidelines for the Evaluation and Management of Heart Failure). *J. Am. Coll. Cardiol.* **46:** 1116–1143.

9. Neuhauser, D. 2002. Ernest Amory Codman MD. *Quality Safety Health Care* **11:** 104–105.

10. Jencks, S.F. & G.R. Wilensky. 1992. The health care quality improvement initiative. A new approach to quality assurance in Medicare. *JAMA* **268:** 900–903.

11. Ellerbeck, E.F. *et al.* 1995. Quality of care for Medicare patients with acute myocardial infarction. A four-state pilot study from the Cooperative Cardiovascular Project. *JAMA* **273:** 1509–1514.

12. Marciniak, T.A. *et al.* 1998. Improving the quality of care for Medicare patients with acute myocardial infarction: results from the Cooperative Cardiovascular Project. *JAMA* **279:** 1351–1357.

13. Grover, F.L., K.E. Hammermeister & C. Burchfiel. 1990. Initial report of the Veterans Administration Preoperative Risk Assessment Study for Cardiac Surgery. *Ann. Thorac. Surg.* **50:** 12–26.

14. Grover, F.L. *et al.* 1994. The Veterans Affairs Continuous Improvement in Cardiac Surgery Study. *Ann. Thorac. Surg.* **58:** 1845–1851.

15. Krumholz, H.M. *et al.* 1997. Quality of care for elderly patients hospitalized with heart failure. *Arch. Intern. Med.* **157:** 2242–2247.

16. Masoudi, F.A. *et al.* 2000. The National Heart Failure Project: a health care financing administration initiative to improve the care of Medicare beneficiaries with heart failure. *Congest. Heart Failure* **6:** 337–339.

17. Havranek, E.P. *et al.* 2002. Spectrum of heart failure in older patients: results from the National Heart Failure project. *Am. Heart J.* **143:** 412–417.

18. Fonarow, G.C. & E.D. Peterson. 2009. Heart failure performance measures and outcomes: real or illusory gains. *JAMA* **302:** 792–794.

19. Donabedian, A. 1966. Evaluating the quality of medical care. *Milbank Memorial Fund Quart.* **44**(Supp l): 166–206.

20. Ross, J.S. *et al.* Hospital volume and 30-day mortality for three common medical conditions. *N. Engl. J. Med.* **362:** 1110–1118.

21. Spertus, J.A. *et al.* 2005. American College of Cardiology and American Heart Association methodology for the selection and creation of performance measures for quantifying the quality of cardiovascular care. *Circulation* **111:** 1703–1712.

22. Spertus, J.A. *et al.* 2010. ACCF/AHA new insights into the methodology of performance measurement. *J. Am. Coll. Cardiol.* **56:** 1767–1782.

23. Bonow, R.O. *et al.* 2008. ACC/AHA classification of care metrics: performance measures and quality metrics. a report of the American College of Cardiology/American Heart Association Task Force on Performance Measures. *J. Am. Coll. Cardiol.* **52:** 2113–2117.

24. ACCF/AHA/PCPI. 2010. American College of Cardiology (ACCF)/American Heart Association (AHA)/Physician Consortium for Performance Improvement (PCPI) Heart Failure Performance Measure Set. www.ama-assn.org/ama1/pub/upload/mm/pcpi/hfset-12-5.pdf. Accessed 26 Dec 2011.

25. Krumholz, H.M. *et al.* 2000. Evaluating quality of care for patients with heart failure. *Circulation* **101:** E122–E140.

26. Masoudi, F.A. *et al.* 2004. National patterns of use and effectiveness of angiotensin-converting enzyme inhibitors in older patients with heart failure and left ventricular systolic dysfunction. *Circulation* **110:** 724–731.

27. The Joint Commission. 2011. Improving America's Hospitals: The Joint Commission's Annual Report on Quality and Safety 2011. Chicago, IL. http://www.jointcommission.org/2011'annual'report/. Accessed 26 Dec 2011.

28. Fonarow, G.C. *et al.* 2007. Association between performance measures and clinical outcomes for patients hospitalized with heart failure. *JAMA* **297:** 61–70.

29. Patterson, M.E. *et al.* 2010. Process of care performance measures and long-term outcomes in patients hospitalized with heart failure. *Med. Care* **48:** 210–216.

30. Hernandez, A.F. *et al.* 2010. Relationships between emerging measures of heart failure processes of care and clinical outcomes. *Am. Heart J.* **159:** 406–413.

31. Werner, R.M. & E.T. Bradlow. 2006. Relationship between Medicare's hospital compare performance measures and mortality rates. *JAMA* **296:** 2694–2702.

32. Krumholz, H.M. *et al.* 2006. An administrative claims model suitable for profiling hospital performance based on 30-day mortality rates among patients with heart failure. *Circulation* **113:** 1693–1701.

33. Krumholz, H.M. *et al.* 2009. Patterns of hospital performance in acute myocardial infarction and heart failure 30-day mortality and readmission. *Circ. Cardiovasc. Qual. Outcomes* **2:** 407–413.

34. Medicare Payment Advisory Commission. 2007. Report to the Congress: promoting greater efficiency in Medicare. www.medpac.gov/documents/jun07'entirereport.pdf. Accessed 26 Dec 2011.

35. Krumholz, H.M. *et al.* 2006. Standards for statistical models used for public reporting of health outcomes: an American Heart Association Scientific Statement from the Quality of Care and Outcomes Research Interdisciplinary Writing Group. Cosponsored by the Council on Epidemiology and Prevention and the Stroke Council Endorsed by the American College of Cardiology Foundation. *Circulation* **113:** 456–462.

36. Krumholz, H.M. *et al.* 2007. Measuring performance for treating heart attacks and heart failure: the case for outcomes measurement. *Health Aff (Millwood)* **26:** 75–85.

37. Bueno, H. *et al.* 2010. Trends in length of stay and short-term outcomes among Medicare patients hospitalized for heart failure, 1993–2006. *JAMA* **303:** 2141–2147.

38. Peterson, E.D. *et al.* 2010. ACCF/AHA 2010 position statement on composite measures for healthcare performance assessment: a report of the American College of Cardiology Foundation/American Heart Association Task Force on Performance Measures (Writing Committee to develop a position statement on composite measures). *Circulation* **121:** 1780–1791.

39. Hernandez, A.F. *et al.* 2011. The need for multiple measures of hospital quality: results from the Get with the Guidelines

heart failure registry of the American Heart Association. *Circulation* **124:** 712–719.

40. Bufalino, V.J. *et al.* 2011. The American Heart Association's recommendations for expanding the applications of existing and future clinical registries: a policy statement from the American Heart Association. *Circulation* **123:** 2167–2179.

41. Radford, M.J. *et al.* 2005. ACC/AHA key data elements and definitions for measuring the clinical management and outcomes of patients with chronic heart failure: a report of the American College of Cardiology/American Heart Association Task Force on Clinical Data Standards (Writing Committee to Develop Heart Failure Clinical Data Standards): developed in collaboration with the American College of Chest Physicians and the International Society for Heart and Lung Transplantation: endorsed by the Heart Failure Society of America. *Circulation* **112:** 1888–1916.

42. Abraham, W.T. *et al.* 2005. In-hospital mortality in patients with acute decompensated heart failure requiring intravenous vasoactive medications: an analysis from the Acute Decompensated Heart Failure National Registry (ADHERE). *J. Am. Coll. Cardiol.* **46:** 57–64.

43. Fonarow, G.C. *et al.* 2004. Organized Program to Initiate Lifesaving Treatment in Hospitalized Patients with Heart Failure (OPTIMIZE-HF): rationale and design. *Am. Heart J.* **148:** 43–51.

44. American Heart Association. 2011. The guideline advantage. http://www.guidelineadvantage.org/TGA/. Accessed 26 Dec 2011.

45. Fonarow, G.C. *et al.* 2010. Improving evidence-based care for heart failure in outpatient cardiology practices: primary results of the Registry to Improve the Use of Evidence-Based Heart Failure Therapies in the Outpatient Setting (IMPROVE HF). *Circulation* **122:** 585–596.

46. US Department of Health & Human Services. 2010. Hospital compare. http://www.hospitalcompare.hss.gov. Accessed 26 Dec 2011.

47. Centers for Medicare and Medicaid Services. 2011. Medicare program; hospital inpatient value-based purchasing program. www.gpo.gov/fdsys/pkg/FR-2011-05-06/pdf/2011-10568.pdf. Accessed 26 Dec 2011.

48. American College of Cardiology Foundation. 2011. The PINNACLE Registry, Vol. 2011.

49. Porter, M.E. 2009. A strategy for health care reform—toward a value-based system. *N. Engl. J. Med.* **361:** 109–112.

50. Porter, M.E. 2010. What is value in health care? *N. Engl. J. Med.* **363:** 2477–2481.

51. Fonarow, G.C. *et al.* 2011. Associations between outpatient heart failure process-of-care measures and mortality. *Circulation* **123:** 1601–1610.

52. Al-Khatib, S.M. *et al.* 2011. Non-evidence-based ICD implantations in the United States. *JAMA* **305:** 43–49.

53. Krumholz, H.M., *et al.* 2008. Standards for measures used for public reporting of efficiency in health care: a scientific statement from the American Heart Association Interdisciplinary Council on Quality of Care and Outcomes research and the American College of Cardiology Foundation. *J. Am. Coll. Cardiol.* **52:** 1518–1526.

54. Pitt, B. *et al.* 1999. The effect of spironolactone on morbidity and mortality in patients with severe heart failure. Randomized Aldactone Evaluation Study Investigators. *N. Engl. J. Med.* **341:** 709–717.

55. Masoudi, F.A. *et al.* 2005. Adoption of spironolactone therapy for older patients with heart failure and left ventricular systolic dysfunction in the United States, 1998–2001. *Circulation* **112:** 39–47.

56. Juurlink, D.N. *et al.* 2004. Rates of hyperkalemia after publication of the randomized aldactone evaluation study. *N. Engl. J. Med.* **351:** 543–551.

57. Masoudi, F.A. *et al.* 2003. Most hospitalized older persons do not meet the enrollment criteria for clinical trials in heart failure. *Am. Heart J.* **146:** 250–257.

58. Rathore, S.S., et al, et al. 2003. Race, quality of care, and outcomes of elderly patients hospitalized with heart failure. *JAMA* **289:** 2517–2524.

59. Chen, J. *et al.* 2011. National and regional trends in heart failure hospitalization and mortality rates for Medicare beneficiaries, 1998–2008. *JAMA* **306:** 1669–1678.

60. Goodlin, S.J. *et al.* 2004. Consensus statement: palliative and supportive care in advanced heart failure. *J. Card. Failure* **10:** 200–209.

Ann. N.Y. Acad. Sci. ISSN 0077-8923

ANNALS OF THE NEW YORK ACADEMY OF SCIENCES
Issue: *Evolving Challenges in Promoting Cardiovascular Health*

Atrial fibrillation, stroke, and quality of life

Jason S. Chinitz,[1,2] Jose M. Castellano,[1,2] Jason C. Kovacic,[1,2] and Valentin Fuster[1,2,3]

[1]Zena and Michael A. Wiener Cardiovascular Institute, [2]Marie-Josée and Henry R. Kravis Cardiovascular Health Center, Mount Sinai School of Medicine, New York, New York. [3]Centro Nacional de Investigaciones Cardiovasculares (CNIC), Madrid, Spain

Address for correspondence: Valentin Fuster, M.D., Ph.D., Zena and Michael A. Wiener Cardiovascular Institute, Mount Sinai Medical Center, One Gustave L. Levy Place, Box 1030, New York, NY 10029-6574. valentin.fuster@mountsinai.org

Contemporary management of atrial fibrillation imposes many challenges, particularly in the setting of our aging population. In addition to well-recognized consequences, such as stroke and mortality, emerging evidence relates atrial fibrillation to elevated risk of dementia, posing further therapeutic challenges. As the incidence of atrial fibrillation rises with age, the balance of controlling stroke risk and limiting major hemorrhage on anticoagulation has become increasingly critical in elderly patients. Appreciation of more extensive risk factors has made it possible to identify patients at very low risk of thromboembolism and higher risk of bleeding. However, practice guidelines in the United States and abroad have occasionally divergent viewpoints regarding how to best manage patients in various risk strata. Options for stroke prevention have expanded with novel antithrombotics and promising mechanical alternatives to anticoagulation, which may be at least as effective in preventing stroke without increasing bleeding risk. Catheter ablation has demonstrated impressive success at preventing atrial fibrillation recurrence in selected patients, and has the potential to further improve outcomes. In addition, the role of antiplatelet medications in patients deemed unsuitable for anticoagulation has been better clarified, although novel agents require further study to assess their impact on thromboembolism. High-bleeding risks associated with the concomitant use of multiple antithrombotics remains a major obstacle in patients with indications for both antiplatelet and anticoagulant therapy.

Keywords: atrial fibrillation; stroke; quality of life; thromboembolism

Introduction

Atrial fibrillation (AF) is the most common sustained cardiac arrhythmia, occurring in 1–2% of the general population. It affects an estimated 2.3 million people in the United States[1] and over 6 million in Europe.[2] The incidence of AF is known to increase exponentially with age,[3] and its prevalence is projected to at least double over the next 50 years with the aging population.[4]

AF is associated with substantial morbidity, including a fivefold increased risk of ischemic stroke,[5] regardless of whether the arrhythmia is paroxysmal, persistent, or permanent.[6] Importantly, AF-related stroke confers increased mortality and greater disability compared to non-AF causes of stroke, including longer hospital stays and lower rates of functional independence after discharge.[5] The risk

of stroke in an individual patient varies based on age and other comorbidities, and accurate assessment of stroke risk can aid in the selection of an appropriate antithrombotic regimen. AF has also been shown to be an independent predictor of mortality,[7] and thus far, only anticoagulation has been shown to reduce AF-related deaths.

Challenge of different perspectives: European and American guidelines

The most widely recognized model for stroke risk assessment, and the one adopted by U.S. guidelines, is the CHADS$_2$ score. The CHADS$_2$ model uses a simple and easily remembered scoring system that assigns points for the presence of various patient risk factors (Table 1A). According to the updated ACCF/AHA/HRS guidelines,[8] patients with

doi: 10.1111/j.1749-6632.2012.06494.x

Ann. N.Y. Acad. Sci. 1254 (2012) 140–150 © 2012 New York Academy of Sciences.

Table 1A. CHADS$_2$ score for stroke risk stratification in patients with nonvalvular atrial fibrillation

CHADS$_2$ risk factor	Score
Congestive heart failure	1
Hypertension	1
Age >75	1
Diabetes mellitus	1
Prior stroke or TIA	2
Maximum score	6

nonvalvular AF and a CHADS$_2$ score of 0 are at low risk of thromboembolism and should be treated with aspirin or no antithrombotic therapy, whereas those with a score of ≥2 are at higher risk and should be treated with anticoagulation. For patients at intermediate risk (CHADS$_2$ score =1), a decision between aspirin or anticoagulation should be based on assessment of the patient's bleeding risk and ability to sustain anticoagulation, and their individual values and preference.

Unfortunately, the CHADS$_2$ score has only fair ability to separate patients into categories corresponding to different rates of thromboembolism. In the ATRIA study, which evaluated a cohort of 13,559 patients with AF off anticoagulation, patients with and without thromboembolism had highly overlapping risk distributions using the CHADS$_2$ model.[9] A recent systematic review and meta-analysis found no significant difference in stroke rates across various risk strata and concluded that the CHADS$_2$ score has minimal clinical utility in predicting ischemic stroke.[6] Undoubtedly, this scheme is insufficient and fails to adequately identify patients at true low risk who may safely avoid anticoagulation. Furthermore, a large proportion of patients fall into the intermediate risk category of CHADS$_2$, leaving management ambiguous.[10] Limitations of the CHADS$_2$ model include its failure to account for the increase in risk with age as a continuous variable, and its exclusion of other previously underappreciated risk factors. The 2006 ACC/AHA/ESC guidelines recommended consideration of "less-validated or weaker risk factors," such as age 65–74, female gender, coronary artery disease, and thyrotoxicosis, when making decisions on antithrombotic therapy.[1]

To be more inclusive of various stroke risk factors, the 2010 European Society of Cardiology (ESC)

Guidelines for the management of AF recommend the use of a newer model, known as CHA$_2$DS$_2$-VASc. This score was derived to complement CHADS$_2$ in decision making and includes the use of additional stroke risk factors, such as age 65–74, female gender, and vascular disease (Table 1B). Numerous validation studies have now shown that the CHA$_2$DS$_2$-VASc score is consistently better than CHADS$_2$ in defining low-risk patients and is at least as good as CHADS$_2$ in defining patients at high stroke risk.[2] In a large Danish registry of 73,538 patients, one-year rates of thromboembolism for patients at lowest risk (score = 0) were 0.78 per 100 person-years under CHA$_2$DS$_2$-VASc and 1.67 per 100 person-years with CHADS$_2$. Using CHA$_2$DS$_2$VASc, this study demonstrated that rates of thromboembolism were lowered with anticoagulation in all risk categories except those with a score of 0. In addition, among patients at intermediate risk based on CHADS$_2$ score = 1, 92.7% were at higher risk based on CHA$_2$DS$_2$VASc.[11]

The assessment of bleeding risk on antithrombotic therapy is vital to management decisions regarding anticoagulation, particularly when stroke risk is intermediate. The HAS-BLED bleeding risk score was derived from multivariate analysis of predictors of bleeding in several cohorts of anticoagulated patients with AF. The HAS-BLED score assigns points for hypertension, abnormal renal or liver function, stroke, bleeding history or predisposition, labile international normalized ratio (INR), age >65 years, and drug or alcohol use. Increasing HAS-BLED scores correlate with a stepwise increment in major bleeding.[10] This model is relatively easy to apply, and performed better than others developed previously. The recent ESC guidelines support use of HAS-BLED, and advice caution when the score is ≥3, including regular patient review.[2]

Although these advanced risk scores were not incorporated into the 2011 ACCF/AHA/HRS guidelines, the CHA$_2$DS$_2$VASc score and HAS-BLED risk models have additive value in identifying patients at low risk for thromboembolism and high risk of bleeding, in whom anticoagulation can be safely deferred. U.S. guidelines recommend the use of aspirin for patients with lone AF, and consideration of aspirin alone for those at intermediate risk even when advanced age is the only risk factor.[8] In contrast, the European guidelines recommend oral anticoagulation for all patients with AF, except in those at lowest

Table 1B. CHA$_2$DS$_2$VASc score for thromboembolic risk stratification in patients with nonvalvular atrial fibrillation

CHA$_2$DS$_2$VASc risk factor	Score
Congestive heart failure/LV dysfunction	1
Hypertension	1
Age $\geq$75	2
Diabetes mellitus	1
Stroke/TIA/thromboembolism	2
Vascular disease	1
Age 65–74	1
Sex category (i.e., female sex)	1
Maximum score	9

risk (CHA$_2$DS$_2$VASc = 0, age < 65 years) or with contraindications to anticoagulation (Table 1C).[2]

Another notable distinction in recent European guidelines involves the use of a symptom severity scale to help guide the decision whether to pursue rhythm control. The presence of symptoms related to AF should be a major factor influencing the decision to attempt restoration of sinus rhythm; however, symptoms are subjective, leaving vague the threshold at which AF becomes unacceptable for a given patient. The 2010 ESC guidelines suggest use of the European Heart Rhythm Association (EHRA) scoring system to assist in this decision-making process (Table 2). The EHRA score intends to consider only symptoms attributable to AF that are likely to improve upon restoration of sinus rhythm or with effective rate control. The ESC guidelines suggest that rate control is a reasonable strategy, particularly in elderly patients, when symptoms related to AF are acceptable (EHRA score $\leq$2); however, patients with higher EHRA scores warrant attempts to restore sinus rhythm.[2]

AF and the brain: beyond stroke

Evidence is emerging that AF contributes to the development of dementia.[12–14] AF is known to increase the risk of stroke, which may result in vascular dementia. The association between AF and cognitive dysfunction, however, has demonstrated broader implications. In the Adult Changes in Thought (ACT) study,[15] a prospective, well-designed population-based cohort study, patients with AF were at higher risk of all-cause demen-

tia (Hazard ratio [HR] 1.34, 95% CI 1.05–1.71) and Alzheimer's dementia (HR 1.41, 95% CI 1.07–1.86) than those without AF, after adjustment for various risk factors, including stroke. In another prospective study of 37,025 patients, those with AF had a higher incidence of all subtypes of dementia (Fig. 1), and among patients who developed dementia, cognitive decline occurred earlier and mortality was higher in patients with AF.[12]

Several biological mechanisms have been proposed to explain the association between AF and dementia. In addition to clinically recognized stroke, patients with AF experience silent cerebral emboli. Although cerebral microinfarcts are an important neuropathological predictor of clinical dementia,[16] it is not known whether AF increases the risk of these microinfarcts. In addition, patients with AF may be predisposed to cerebral hypoperfusion as a result of heart rate variability and comorbid heart failure.[17] These vascular insults may act synergistically with other neuropathological processes common in patients with late-life dementia, such as neurofibrillary tangles, Lewy bodies, and hippocampal sclerosis, to lower cognitive reserves and accelerate the onset of cognitive decline.[18]

AF and nonvascular types of dementia may also share common underlying risk factors and pathophysiologic mechanisms, such as inflammation. In patients with elevated markers of systemic inflammation, there is increased long-term risk all-cause dementia.[19] Similarly, AF is associated with elevated biomarkers of inflammation, independent of other cardiac risk factors.[20] Activation of a chronic inflammatory response associated with both AF and dementia may accelerate cerebral microvascular dysfunction and other causes of neuronal injury, resulting in impaired cerebral perfusion and progressive cognitive decline. Finally, the presence of dementia may also predispose to the development of AF through neurologic changes that alter autonomic input to the heart.

The association between AF and dementia has important clinical implications given the high prevalence of AF and the substantial burden imposed by dementia on patients and their families. However, it is not yet known whether various treatments for AF can modify the risk or timing of incident dementia in an individual patient. A recent nonrandomized observational study reported a lower risk of dementia in patients with AF who underwent

Table 1C. Comparison between anticoagulation recommendations in the ACC/AHA/HRS[33] and ESC guidelines[2]

Stroke risk	ACCF/AHA/HRS guidelines	ESC guidelines
Low risk	$CHADS_2 = 0$	$CHA_2DS_2VASc = 0$
	Aspirin recommended	Prefer no anticoagulation over aspirin
Moderate risk	$CHADS_2 = 1$	$CHA_2DS_2VASc = 1$
	Oral anticoagulation or Aspirin recommended	Prefer oral anticoagulation over aspirin
High risk	$CHADS_2 > 2$	$CHA_2DS_2VASc > 2$
	Oral anticoagulation recommended	Oral anticoagulation recommended

catheter ablation.[21] Additional research is needed to examine the relationship between AF and cognitive decline, and to determine whether specific treatment strategies for AF, such as anticoagulation or restoration of sinus rhythm, can modify cognitive outcomes.

Challenge of international normalized ratio

Vitamin K antagonists (VKAs), such as warfarin, are highly effective in decreasing the risk of AF-related stroke. Compared to placebo, VKAs are associated with a 67% relative risk reduction[22] and provide a 40% relative risk reduction compared to aspirin.[23] Unfortunately, VKAs have several limitations, including a narrow therapeutic index, frequent food and drug interactions, and the need for regular monitoring of anticoagulation intensity. Even in carefully monitored settings, it is often difficult to maintain the international normalized ratio (INR) within target range (typical goal INR 2–3); in a meta-analysis, the proportion of time INR was in the therapeutic range in patients treated with VKAs averaged 65% in clinical trials and only 56% in retrospective studies.[24] Fortunately, small improvements in therapeutic time can have a substantial impact on clinical outcome. In the same meta-analysis a 10% increase in time within therapeutic range was associated with a 1% lower annual rate of thromboembolic events, and an even larger reduction in major hemorrhage.[24] Among 5,791 patients randomized to the warfarin arm of the multicenter Randomized Evaluation of Long-Term Anticoagulation Therapy (RE-LY) trial, total events, including thromboembolism and major bleeding, were lowest when the INR was within therapeutic range over 72.6% of the time; however, even in this carefully controlled trial, the mean time within therapeutic range achieved in centers within the Unites States averaged 66%.[25]

Regulated systems for self-management of anticoagulation intensity, allowing patients to monitor and adjust their own warfarin dosing, are economically attractive and have the potential improve outcomes. In one study, use of a physician-supervised internet-based self-management protocol increased time within therapeutic range from 63% to 74% compared to a standard anticoagulation management clinic.[26] A recent meta-analysis revealed a 49% relative risk reduction in thromboembolic events with self-monitoring systems compared to standard management, with particularly impressive results in patients younger than 55 years of age.[27]

Challenge of age

The risk of stroke in patients with AF increases with age, as does the risk of bleeding on anticoagulation, raising controversy regarding optimal management in older patients. However, the benefit of anticoagulation increases substantially in patients with higher absolute stroke risks, including those with advanced age, whereas the harm increases only moderately. Without anticoagulation, the two-year incidence of stroke in the Framingham Heart Study increased steadily from 5.5% in patients aged 50–59 years to 14.3% in octogenarians.[28] In comparison, the risk of intracranial hemorrhage on warfarin therapy increases 2.5-fold in patients 85 years of age or older.[29] A cohort study found the net clinical benefit of anticoagulation (rate of stroke prevented by warfarin relative to rate of intracranial hemorrhage on warfarin) to rise steadily with age and was highest for those 85 years or older (Fig. 2).[30] The net clinical benefit favoring anticoagulation persisted even when intracranial hemorrhage was given a severity weighting factor of 1.5 to 2 times that of stroke, highlighting the importance of effective stroke

Table 2. European Society of Cardiology guidelines for classification of symptoms related to atrial fibrillation

EHRA score	
EHRA class	Explanation
EHRA I	No symptoms
EHRA II	Mild symptoms, normal daily life not affected
EHRA III	Severe symptoms, normal daily life affected
EHRA IV	Disabling symptoms, normal daily activity discontinued

EHRA, European Heart Rhythm Association.

prevention despite elevated bleeding risk in the elderly.

Challenge of novel platelet inhibitors

Dual-antiplatelet therapy as a potential alternative to warfarin for stroke prevention in patients with AF was evaluated in the ACTIVE-W (Atrial Fibrillation Clopidogrel Trial with Irbesartan for Prevention of Vascular Events) study, in which patients with an average of two stroke risk factors were randomized to aspirin + clopidogrel or a VKA, open-label. The primary outcome of stroke, embolism, myocardial infarction, or vascular death occurred less often in the VKA group (3.9 vs. 5.6%/year, relative risk 1.44, $P = 0.0003$), and total adverse outcomes, including bleeding, were more frequent in patients randomized to aspirin + clopidogrel (relative risk 1.41, $P < 0.001$).[31] The ACTIVE-A trial evaluated aspirin alone versus dual-antiplatelet therapy in patients deemed unsuitable for anticoagulation. The dual-antiplatelet combination was associated with a 28% lower rate of stroke (2.4 vs. 3.3%/year, $P < 0.001$), but a higher rate of major bleeding (2.0 vs. 1.3%/year, $P < 0.001$).[32] Addition of clopidogrel to aspirin might be considered for patients with AF when anticoagulation with warfarin is considered unsuitable (Class IIb recommendation).[33]

The development of safer and more effective antiplatelet agents, although not yet studied for stroke prevention in AF, has the potential to further increase management options. Ticagrelor, a novel antiplatelet agent that provides greater antagonism of the adenosine diphosphate receptor $P2Y_{12}$ than

clopidogrel, demonstrated similar rates of major bleeding compared to clopidogrel with greater efficacy in patients with acute coronary syndromes.[34] Recently, a novel class of antiplatelet agents that inhibit thrombin-mediated platelet activation, including vorapaxar and E-5555 (atopaxar), have sparked interest in their potential to improve ischemic outcomes without significantly increasing bleeding liability.[35] In a Phase II study of patients with high-risk coronary artery disease or acute coronary syndromes, E-5555 added to standard antiplatelet therapy did not increase clinically significant bleeding, although there was a higher rate of any TIMI bleeding with the highest dosage and a dose-dependent increase in liver function test abnormalities and QTc interval.[36] The efficacy of these agents in patients with AF, as well as their safety in combination with other antithrombotics, will require careful study as these novel agents become more widely used.

Challenge of multiple antithrombotics

The concomitant use of multiple antithrombotics is associated with particularly high bleeding risk. In clinical practice, such combinations are frequently considered given the common coexistence of AF with coronary artery disease and associated percutaneous coronary intervention (PCI) obliging treatment with dual-antiplatelet therapy. Antiplatelet agents alone may provide sufficient protection from thromboembolism in patients with AF at lower stroke risk ($CHADS_2$ score 0–1); however, in higher

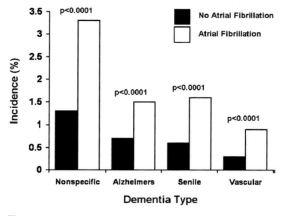

Figure 1. Increased incidence of various subtypes of dementia in patients with atrial fibrillation. Reproduced with permission from Elsevier Limited.[12]

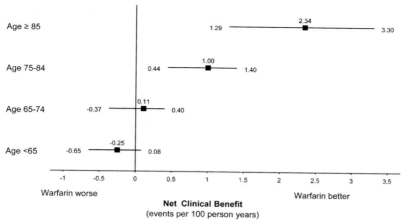

Figure 2. The net clinical benefit of warfarin by age group, with intracranial hemorrhage weighted as 1.5 times the value of thromboembolism. Net clinical benefit is defined as the annualized rate of thromboembolic events prevented minus the annualized rate of intracranial hemorrhage induced by warfarin therapy. Horizontal bars represent 95% confidence intervals. Reproduced with permission from the American College of Physicians.[30]

risk patients, consideration of "triple therapy" (warfarin + aspirin + clopidogrel) is necessary after PCI. In a meta-analysis of 10 studies involving 1,349 patients receiving triple therapy, the incidence of major bleeding was 2.2% (95% CI 0.7–3.7%) at only 30 days.[37] Another meta-analysis demonstrated the relative risk of major bleeding to be four times higher with triple therapy than with a dual-antiplatelet regimen.[38]

As the incremental benefit of clopidogrel in addition to aspirin after PCI is time-limited, the duration of treatment with triple antithrombotic therapy should be as short as possible. In a prospective cohort study of 6,816 patients receiving implantation of a drug-eluting stent, most episodes of stent thrombosis occurred early after PCI, and no substantial protective effect of clopidogrel in addition to aspirin was demonstrated after the first six months.[39] Similarly, the incremental bleeding risk associated with the addition of clopidogrel to aspirin appears concentrated in the first year of treatment.[40] As stent thrombosis is associated with high mortality rates, triple therapy may still be warranted in patients with AF at moderate-to-high stroke risk ($CHADS_2 > 1$) after PCI, although the duration should be limited to no more than one month for patients receiving bare metal stents, and six months for those receiving drug-eluting stents. Thereafter, treatment with warfarin and aspirin alone is advisable.[38]

Challenge of novel anticoagulants

In October 2010, dabigatran etexilate, an oral direct thrombin inhibitor that does not require routine monitoring of anticoagulation intensity, gained FDA approval. The RE-LY trial compared two doses to warfarin, and found that dabigatran 150 mg twice daily reduced the stroke rate by 34% (1.11 vs. 1.71%/year, superiority $P < 0.001$) with no increase in major bleeding. Dabigatran reduced the rate of hemorrhagic stroke compared to warfarin (0.11 vs. 0.38%/year, $P < 0.001$), and there was a trend toward reduced mortality (3.64 vs. 4.13%/year, $P = 0.051$).[41] A marginally increased risk of myocardial infarction was seen with dabigatran (0.81 vs. 0.64%/year; $P = 0.12$), as well as a higher rate of gastrointestinal bleeding, and dyspepsia (in approximately 10% of patients). Limitations of dabigatran include the lack of an antidote and drug accumulation in patients with renal insufficiency. Lower dose dabigatran (110 mg twice daily) yielded stroke rates noninferior to those with warfarin with lower rates of major hemorrhage, but this dose was not approved. Another dose of dabigatran, 75 mg twice daily, was approved but has not been well studied. Questions remain regarding optimal dosing in elderly patients and those at lower thromboembolic risk. The ACCF/AHA/HRS revised guidelines recommend dabigatran for stroke-prone patients with AF without prosthetic heart valves, rheumatic

Table 3. Clinical trials of new anticoagulants

	Dabigatran RELY, $n = 18{,}113$	Rivaroxaban ROCKET-AF, $n = 14{,}264$	Apixaban AVERROES, $n = 5{,}600$	Apixaban ARISTOTLE, $n = 18{,}201$
Type	Noninferiority	Noninferiority	Superiority	Noninferiority
Study drugs	Dabigatran 150 mg bid Dabigatran 110 mg bid Warfarin (INR2–3)	Rivaroxaban 20 mg qd Warfarin (INR2–3)	Apixaban 5 mg bid Aspirin 81–324 mg qd	Apixaban 5 mg bid Warfarin (INR2–3)
Other doses	None. 75 mg bid (unstudied) was approved by FDA for CrCl 15–30 mL/min	15 mg qd in patients with CrCl 30–49 mL/min	2.5 mg bid in patients with two criteria: age ≥ 80 years, weight ≤ 60 kg, Cr > 1.5 mg/dL	
Stroke risk	Moderate–high risk $CHADS_2 > 1$	Moderate–high risk $CHADS_2 > 2$	Moderate–high risk $CHADS_2 > 1$	Moderate–high risk $CHADS_2 > 1$
Primary efficacy outcome	9% reduction in stroke or systemic embolism for 110 mg, 34% reduction for 150 mg ($P < 0.001$ for both)	21% reduction in stroke or systemic embolism ($P < 0.001$)	55% reduction in stroke or systemic embolism ($P < 0.001$)	21% reduction in stroke or systemic embolism (noninferiority $P < 0.001$)
Safety outcome	20% reduction in major bleeding for 110 mg ($P = 0.003$), no difference for 150 mg	No difference in major and clinically relevant nonmajor bleeding ($P = 0.44$)	No difference in major bleeding ($P = 0.57$)	31% reduction in major bleeding ($P < 0.001$)

bid, twice daily; CrCl, creatinine clearance; dl, deciliter; FDA, Food and Drug Administration; INR, international normalized ratio; kg, kilogram; mg, milligram; qd, once daily.

heart disease, renal failure, or advanced liver disease (Class I).[33]

Oral factor Xa inhibitors have also shown promise as anticoagulants for stroke prevention in patients with AF. In the Rivaroxaban Once Daily Oral Direct Factor Xa Inhibitor Compared with Vitamin K Antagonism for Prevention of Stroke and Embolism Trial in Atrial Fibrillation (ROCKET-AF) among 14,264 patients at high risk for thromboembolism (mean $CHADS_2$ score = 3.5), rivaroxaban proved noninferior to warfarin with regard to prevention of stroke and systemic embolism (1.7 vs. 2.2%/year, noninferiority $P < 0.001$). Rates of major bleeding were similar to warfarin (3.4 vs. 3.6%/year, $P = 0.58$), but rivaroxaban-treated patients had significant fewer intracranial hemorrhages (0.5 vs. 0.7%/year, $P = 0.02$) and fatal bleeds (0.2 vs. 0.5%/year, $P = 0.003$).[42] Some patients may prefer the once-daily dosing of rivaroxaban, which was

approved for clinical use by the FDA in November 2011.

Apixaban, another oral factor Xa inhibitor, has demonstrated at least as promising results but has not yet gained FDA approval. In the Apixaban Versus Acetylsalicylic Acid to Prevent Stroke in Atrial Fibrillation Patients Who Have Failed or Are Unsuitable for Vitamin K Antagonist Treatment (AVERROES) trial, apixiban was superior to aspirin in patients with AF unwilling or unsuitable for VKA therapy, without significant difference in rates of major bleeding.[43] In the subsequent Apixaban for Reduction in Stroke and Other Thromboembolic Events in Atrial Fibrillation (ARISTOTLE) trial, twice daily apixaban was compared to warfarin in 18,201 patients with AF and at least one risk factor for stroke (mean $CHADS_2$ score 2.1); after a median follow-up of 1.8 years, apixaban demonstrated superior prevention of stroke or systemic embolism (1.27

vs. 1.60%/year, HR 0.79, superiority $P = 0.01$), less major bleeding (2.13 vs. 3.09%/year, $P < 0.001$), and a 58% relative risk reduction in intracranial hemorrhage (0.33 vs. 0.80%/year, $P < 0.001$). In addition, apixaban was associated with 11% lower all-cause mortality than warfarin ($P = 0.047$).[44] Compared to warfarin, the oral factor Xa inhibitors without routine coagulation monitoring appear at least as effective with more favorable bleeding profiles (Table 3). However, the cost of these agents has not been announced, and effective antidotes are not available.

Challenge of interventional approaches to stroke prevention

On the basis of studies demonstrating that the left atrial appendage is the most important source of thrombi in patients with non-valvular AF,[45] non-pharmacological alternatives for stroke prevention have been developed based on appendage occlusion. In the Watchman Left Atrial Appendage System for Embolic Protection in Patients with AF (PROTECT AF) trial, the Watchman occlusion device percutaneously implanted at the ostium of the left atrial appendage compared favorably to warfarin with regard to the composite endpoint of stroke, cardiovascular or unexplained death, or systemic embolism at a mean follow-up of 18 months. The incidence of the safety endpoint was greater in patients randomized to device implantation, driven predominantly by pericardial effusion and procedure-related ischemic stroke.[46] With extended follow-up, it appears that most complications associated with the device occur in the early postprocedure period and decline with operator experience. The functional impact of adverse effects, an outcome driven by disability or death associated with treatment, may actually favor Watchman implantation over long-term warfarin therapy.[47] Other methods of left atrial appendage closure, such as epicardial suture ligation that do not require periprocedural anticoagulation, are in development.[48,49]

Catheter ablation of AF has the potential to decrease stroke rates by effectively restoring sinus rhythm, but this has not yet been proven. Despite clear associations between AF and stroke, several randomized studies have failed to demonstrate any improvement in stroke risk with a management strategy aimed at restoration of sinus rhythm.[50–55] Presumably, the failure of a rhythm control strategy

to improve long-term outcomes in these trials is in large part due to the limited ability of the antiarrhythmic medications used in them to successfully restore sinus rhythm.[56] Ablation, however, can effectively maintain sinus rhythm in most patients with better long-term safety than antiarrhythmic drugs. In one randomized, multicenter comparison in patients with paroxysmal AF, freedom from symptomatic recurrence over nine months was achieved in 66% of patients after ablation compared to 16% with antiarrhythmic medications ($P < 0.001$), and major 30-day treatment related adverse events were lower after ablation.[57] Other studies have reported one-year success rates around 85% after ablation of paroxysmal AF, albeit with higher rates of recurrence in patients with persistent arrhythmia.[58,59] It is conceivable that when AF is successfully eliminated by ablation, thromboembolic risk may be reduced. In support of this concept, a recent international multicenter registry demonstrated rates of death and stroke to be significantly lower in patients who underwent ablation compared to a separate cohort of patients with medically managed AF from the Euro Heart Survey (stroke rate 0.5% vs. 2.8% per patient-year, $P < 0.0001$); outcomes after ablation in this registry were similar to a hypothetical matched cohort of patients without AF (Fig. 3).[59] Results from ongoing randomized trials are needed

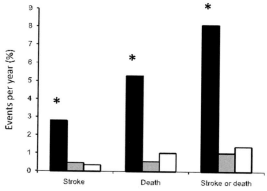

Figure 3. Stroke, death, and combined outcomes after ablation of atrial fibrillation in a multicenter international registry compared with patients treated medically in the Euro Heart Survey, and a hypothetical cohort of matched controls without atrial fibrillation using mortality and stroke rates from UK national statistics. *Indicates a significant difference between the "medical" cohort and the other two groups. Reproduced with permission from BMJ Publishing Group Ltd.[59] *$P < 0.0001$. Black shading, medical; gray shading, ablation; no shading, general population.

to determine whether successful restoration and maintenance of sinus rhythm after AF ablation will correlate with long-term reductions in stroke and mortality.

Conclusion

AF is extremely common and associated with increased mortality and substantial morbidity, including high rates of stroke and dementia. In our aging population, AF has become so prevalent that a thorough understanding of the challenges inherent to various management strategies must be well understood by all clinicians. The field of anticoagulation in AF is rapidly evolving as safer pharmacological alternatives to warfarin, which do not require routine monitoring, and more effective interventional therapies become available. Novel risk scores make it possible to identify patients at very low risk of thromboembolism, in whom anticoagulation may be safely deferred. Patient-specific factors, including bleeding risk, make an individualized approach to antithrombotic therapy critical. Recent European guidelines contribute important perspectives toward this approach and have the potential to improve outcomes for our patients with atrial fibrillation.

Conflicts of interest

The authors declare no conflicts of interest.

References

1. Fuster, V. *et al.* 2006. ACC/AHA/ESC 2006 Guidelines for the management of patients with atrial fibrillation: a report of the American College of Cardiology/American Heart Association Task Force on Practice Guidelines and the European Society of Cardiology Committee for Practice Guidelines (Writing Committee to Revise the 2001 Guidelines for the Management of Patients With Atrial Fibrillation). Developed in collaboration with the European Heart Rhythm Association and the Heart Rhythm Society. *Circulation* **114:** e257–e354.
2. Camm, A.J. *et al.* 2010. Guidelines for the management of atrial fibrillation: the task force for the management of atrial fibrillation of the European Society of Cardiology (ESC). *Eur. Heart J.* **31:** 2369–2429.
3. Friberg, L., N. Hammar & M. Rosenqvist. 2010. Stroke in paroxysmal atrial fibrillation: report from the Stockholm Cohort of Atrial Fibrillation. *Eur. Heart J.* **31:** 967–975.
4. Roger, V.L. *et al.* 2011. Heart disease and stroke statistics–2011 update: a report from the American Heart Association. *Circulation* **123:** e18–e209.
5. Lin, H.J. *et al.* 1996. Stroke severity in atrial fibrillation. The Framingham Study. *Stroke* **27:** 1760–1764.
6. Keogh, C., E. Wallace, C. Dillon, *et al.* 2011. Validation of the CHADS2 clinical prediction rule to predict ischaemic stroke. A systematic review and meta-analysis. *Thromb. Haemost.* **106:** 528–538.
7. Krahn, A.D., J. Manfreda, R.B. Tate, *et al.* 1995. The natural history of atrial fibrillation: incidence, risk factors, and prognosis in the Manitoba Follow-Up Study. *Am. J. Med.* **98:** 476–484.
8. Wann, L.S. *et al.* 2011. 2011 ACCF/AHA/HRS focused update on the management of patients with atrial fibrillation (update on Dabigatran): a report of the American College of Cardiology Foundation/American Heart Association Task Force on practice guidelines. *Circulation* **123:** 1144–1150.
9. Fang, M.C. *et al.* 2008. Comparison of risk stratification schemes to predict thromboembolism in people with non-valvular atrial fibrillation. *J. Am. Coll. Cardiol.* **51:** 810–815.
10. Lip, G.Y. 2011. Implications of the CHA(2)DS(2)-VASc and HAS-BLED Scores for thromboprophylaxis in atrial fibrillation. *Am. J. Med.* **124:** 111–114.
11. Olesen, J.B. *et al.* 2011. Validation of risk stratification schemes for predicting stroke and thromboembolism in patients with atrial fibrillation: nationwide cohort study. *BMJ* **342:** d124.
12. Bunch, T.J. *et al.* 2010. Atrial fibrillation is independently associated with senile, vascular, and Alzheimer's dementia. *Heart Rhythm* **7:** 433–437.
13. Ott, A. *et al.* 1997. Atrial fibrillation and dementia in a population-based study. The Rotterdam Study. *Stroke* **28:** 316–321.
14. Forti, P. *et al.* 2006. Atrial fibrillation and risk of dementia in non-demented elderly subjects with and without mild cognitive impairment. *Neurol. Res.* **28:** 625–629.
15. Dublin, S. *et al.* 2011. Atrial fibrillation and risk of dementia: a prospective cohort study. *J. Am. Geriatr. Soc.* **59:** 1369–1375.
16. Sonnen, J.A. *et al.* 2007. Pathological correlates of dementia in a longitudinal, population-based sample of aging. *Ann. Neurol.* **62:** 406–413.
17. Lavy, S. *et al.* 1980. Effect of chronic atrial fibrillation on regional cerebral blood flow. *Stroke* **11:** 35–38.
18. Fotuhi, M., V. Hachinski & P.J. Whitehouse. 2009. Changing perspectives regarding late-life dementia. *Nat. Rev. Neurol.* **5:** 649–658.
19. Schmidt, R. *et al.* 2002. Early inflammation and dementia: a 25-year follow-up of the Honolulu-Asia Aging Study. *Ann. Neurol.* **52:** 168–174.
20. Crandall, M.A. *et al.* 2009. Atrial fibrillation and CHADS2 risk factors are associated with highly sensitive C-reactive protein incrementally and independently. *Pacin. Clin. Electrophysiol.* **32:** 648–652.
21. Bunch, T.J. *et al.* 2011. Patients treated with catheter ablation for atrial fibrillation have long-term rates of death, stroke, and dementia similar to patients without atrial fibrillation. *J. Cardiovasc. Electrophysiol.* **22:** 839–845.
22. Cairns, J.A. 1991. Stroke prevention in atrial fibrillation trial. *Circulation* **84:** 933–935.
23. Hart, R.G. & J.L. Halperin. 1999. Atrial fibrillation and thromboembolism: a decade of progress in stroke prevention. *Ann. Intern. Med.* **131:** 688–695.
24. Wan, Y. *et al.* 2008. Anticoagulation control and prediction of adverse events in patients with atrial fibrillation:

a systematic review. *Circ. Cardiovasc. Qual. Outcomes* **1**: 84–91.

25. Wallentin, L. *et al.* 2010. Efficacy and safety of dabigatran compared with warfarin at different levels of international normalised ratio control for stroke prevention in atrial fibrillation: an analysis of the RE-LY trial. *Lancet* **376**: 975–983.

26. O'Shea, S.I. *et al.* 2008. Direct-to-patient expert system and home INR monitoring improves control of oral anticoagulation. *J. Thromb. Thrombolysis* **26**: 14–21.

27. Heneghan, C., A. Ward & R. Perera. 2012. Self-monitoring of oral anticoagulation: systematic review and meta-analysis of individual patient data. *Lancet* **379**: 322–334.

28. Wolf, P.A., R.D. Abbott & W.B. Kannel. 1987. Atrial fibrillation: a major contributor to stroke in the elderly. The Framingham Study. *Arch. Intern. Med.* **147**: 1561–1564.

29. Fang, M.C. *et al.* 2004. Advanced age, anticoagulation intensity, and risk for intracranial hemorrhage among patients taking warfarin for atrial fibrillation. *Ann. Intern. Med.* **141**: 745–752.

30. Singer, D.E. *et al.* 2009. The net clinical benefit of warfarin anticoagulation in atrial fibrillation. *Ann. Intern. Med.* **151**: 297–305.

31. Connolly, S. *et al.* 2006. Clopidogrel plus aspirin versus oral anticoagulation for atrial fibrillation in the Atrial fibrillation Clopidogrel Trial with Irbesartan for prevention of vascular events (ACTIVE W): a randomised controlled trial. *Lancet* **367**: 1903–1912.

32. Connolly, S.J. *et al.* 2009. Effect of clopidogrel added to aspirin in patients with atrial fibrillation. *N. Engl. J. Med.* **360**: 2066–2078.

33. Wann, L.S. *et al.* 2011. 2011 ACCF/AHA/HRS focused update on the management of patients with atrial fibrillation (Updating the 2006 Guideline): a report of the American College of Cardiology Foundation/American Heart Association Task Force on Practice Guidelines. *J. Am. Coll. Cardiol.* **57**: 223–242.

34. Wallentin, L. *et al.* 2009. Ticagrelor versus clopidogrel in patients with acute coronary syndromes. *N. Engl. J. Med.* **361**: 1045–1057.

35. Leonardi, S., P. Tricoci & R.C. Becker. 2010. Thrombin receptor antagonists for the treatment of atherothrombosis: therapeutic potential of vorapaxar and E-5555. *Drugs* **70**: 1771–1783.

36. Goto, S., H. Ogawa, M. Takeuchi, *et al.* 2010. Double-blind, placebo-controlled Phase II studies of the protease-activated receptor 1 antagonist E5555 (atopaxar) in Japanese patients with acute coronary syndrome or high-risk coronary artery disease. *Eur. Heart J.* **31**: 2601–2613.

37. Paikin, J.S., D.S. Wright, M.A. Crowther, *et al.* 2010. Triple antithrombotic therapy in patients with atrial fibrillation and coronary artery stents. *Circulation* **121**: 2067–2070.

38. Sourgounis, A., J. Lipiecki, T.S. Lo, & M. Hamon. 2009. Coronary stents and chronic anticoagulation. *Circulation* **119**: 1682–1688.

39. Schulz, S. *et al.* 2009. Stent thrombosis after drug-eluting stent implantation: incidence, timing, and relation to discontinuation of clopidogrel therapy over a 4-year period. *Eur. Heart J.* **30**: 2714–2721.

40. Berger, P.B. *et al.* 2010. Bleeding complications with dual antiplatelet therapy among patients with stable vascular disease or risk factors for vascular disease: results from the Clopidogrel for High Atherothrombotic Risk and Ischemic Stabilization, Management, and Avoidance (CHARISMA) trial. *Circulation* **121**: 2575–2583.

41. Connolly, S.J. *et al.* 2009. Dabigatran versus warfarin in patients with atrial fibrillation. *N. Engl. J. Med.* **361**: 1139–1151.

42. Patel, M.R. *et al.* 2011. Rivaroxaban versus warfarin in nonvalvular atrial fibrillation. *N. Engl. J. Med.* **365**: 883–891.

43. Connolly, S.J. *et al.* 2011. Apixaban in patients with atrial fibrillation. *N. Engl. J. Med.* **364**: 806–817.

44. Granger, C.B., J.H. Alexander, J.J.V. McMurray, *et al.* 2011. Apixaban versus warfarin in patients with atrial fibrillation. *N. Engl. J. Med.* **365**: 981–992.

45. Stoddard, M.F., P.R. Dawkins, C.R. Prince & N.M. Ammash. 1995. Left atrial appendage thrombus is not uncommon in patients with acute atrial fibrillation and a recent embolic event: a transesophageal echocardiographic study. *J. Am. Coll. Cardiol.* **25**: 452–459.

46. Holmes, D.R. *et al.* 2009. Percutaneous closure of the left atrial appendage versus warfarin therapy for prevention of stroke in patients with atrial fibrillation: a randomised non-inferiority trial. *Lancet* **374**: 534–542.

47. Reddy, V.Y., D. Holmes, S.K. Doshi, *et al.* 2011. Safety of percutaneous left atrial appendage closure: results from the Watchman Left Atrial Appendage System for Embolic Protection in Patients with AF (PROTECT AF) clinical trial and the Continued Access Registry. *Circulation* **123**: 417–424.

48. Singh, S.M., S.R. Dukkipati, A. d'Avila, *et al.* 2010. Percutaneous left atrial appendage closure with an epicardial suture ligation approach: a prospective randomized pre-clinical feasibility study. *Heart Rhythm* **7**: 370–376.

49. Bruce, C.J. *et al.* 2011. Percutaneous epicardial left atrial appendage closure: intermediate-term results. *J. Cardiovasc. Electrophysiol.* **22**: 64–70.

50. Wyse, D.G. *et al.* 2002. A comparison of rate control and rhythm control in patients with atrial fibrillation. *N. Engl. J. Med.* **347**: 1825–1833.

51. Van Gelder, I.C. *et al.* 2002. A comparison of rate control and rhythm control in patients with recurrent persistent atrial fibrillation. *N. Engl. J. Med.* **347**: 1834–1840.

52. Hohnloser, S.H., K.H. Kuck & J. Lilienthal. 2000. Rhythm or rate control in atrial fibrillation–Pharmacological intervention in atrial fibrillation (PIAF): a randomised trial. *Lancet* **356**: 1789–1794.

53. Opolski, G. *et al.* 2004. Rate control vs rhythm control in patients with nonvalvular persistent atrial fibrillation: the results of the Polish How to Treat Chronic Atrial Fibrillation (HOT CAFE) Study. *Chest* **126**: 476–486.

54. Carlsson, J. *et al.* 2003. Randomized trial of rate-control versus rhythm-control in persistent atrial fibrillation: the Strategies of Treatment of Atrial Fibrillation (STAF) study. *J. Am. Coll. Cardiol.* **41**: 1690–1696.

55. Roy, D. *et al.* 2008. Rhythm control versus rate control for atrial fibrillation and heart failure. *N. Engl. J. Med.* **358**: 2667–2677.

56. Corley, S.D. *et al.* 2004. Relationships between sinus rhythm, treatment, and survival in the Atrial Fibrillation Follow-Up Investigation of Rhythm Management (AFFIRM) Study. *Circulation* **109:** 1509–1513.

57. Wilber, D.J. *et al.* 2010. Comparison of antiarrhythmic drug therapy and radiofrequency catheter ablation in patients with paroxysmal atrial fibrillation: a randomized controlled trial. *JAMA* **303:** 333–340.

58. Pappone, C. *et al.* 2006. A randomized trial of circumferential pulmonary vein ablation versus antiarrhythmic drug therapy in paroxysmal atrial fibrillation: the APAF Study. *J. Am. Coll. Cardiol.* **48:** 2340–2347.

59. Hunter, R.J. *et al.* 2012. Maintenance of sinus rhythm with an ablation strategy in patients with atrial fibrillation is associated with a lower risk of stroke and death. *Heart* **98:** 48–53.

Ann. N.Y. Acad. Sci. ISSN 0077-8923

ANNALS OF THE NEW YORK ACADEMY OF SCIENCES
Issue: *Evolving Challenges in Promoting Cardiovascular Health*

Transcatheter aortic valve implantation and cerebrovascular events: the current state of the art

Brian G. Hynes and Josep Rodés-Cabau

Quebec Heart and Lung Institute, Laval University, Quebec City, Quebec, Canada

Address for correspondence: Josep Rodés-Cabau, Quebec Heart and Lung Institute, Laval University, 2725 Chemin Ste-Foy, G1V 4G5 Quebec City, Quebec, Canada. josep.rodes@criucpq.ulaval.ca

Transcatheter aortic valve implantation (TAVI) has revolutionized the care of high-risk patients with severe calcific aortic stenosis. Those considered at high or prohibitive risk of major adverse outcomes with open surgical aortic valve replacement may now be offered an alternative less-invasive therapy. Despite the rapid evolution and clinical application of this new technology, recent studies have raised concerns about adverse cerebrovascular event rates in patients undergoing TAVI. In this review, we explore the current data both in relation to procedure-related silent cerebrovascular ischemic events, as well as clinically apparent stroke. The timing of neurological events and their prognostic implications are also examined. Finally, potential mechanisms of TAVI-related cerebrovascular injury are described, in addition to efforts to minimize their occurrence.

Keywords: transcatheter aortic valve implantation; aortic stenosis; stroke

Introduction

Aortic stenosis (AS) represents the most common valvular disorder in both Europe and North America and is estimated to affect up to 2–4% of the elderly population.[1,2] In 2002, Cribier *et al.*[3] detailed the first transcatheter aortic valve implantation (TAVI) in a 57-year-old man with calcific AS. The rapid clinical expansion of TAVI has established a paradigm shift in the management of patients with severe aortic valve stenosis.[4] Patients deemed to be at prohibitively high-risk of adverse outcomes with open surgical aortic valve replacement (SAVR), may now be assessed for suitability for valve replacement employing a less invasive approach. However, recent data have raised concerns in relation to the risk of TAVI-related stroke.[5] In this review, we will detail the current information pertaining to TAVI, with a particular emphasis on the associated adverse cerebrovascular events. Although new TAVI systems are in a continuous state of development, two TAVI devices— the balloon-expandable Edwards valve (Edwards Lifesciences California) and the self-expandable CoreValve ReValving (Medtronic)—have been used

most extensively and will form the basis of this review. Both valve systems and associated procedural details have been described elsewhere.[4]

Cerebral ischemic defects following TAVI

Recently, the issue of clinically silent cerebrovascular insults associated with TAVI has come to the fore following a series of studies evaluating cerebral ischemic events using diffusion-weighted magnetic resonance imaging (DW MRI; Table 1, Figs. 1 and 2). Kahlert *et al.*[6] compared 32 patients undergoing transfemoral (TF) TAVI (22 with the Edwards Sapien valve and 18 with the CoreValve) with historical SAVR controls ($n = 21$; Table 1). Patients underwent DW MRI at baseline, a mean of 3.4 (2.5–4.4) days and again at three months after the index procedure. In addition, all patients were assessed by an experienced neurologist using the National Institutes of Health Stroke Scale (NIHSS) and the Mini-Mental State Examination (MMSE). Successful valve implantation was achieved in all TAVI patients with no obvious adverse neurologic events during the periprocedural period. No change was noted in the NIHSS scale or MMSE score of any of these patients. Repeat DW MRI post-TAVI,

doi: 10.1111/j.1749-6632.2012.06477.x

Table 1. DW MRI studies post-TAVI

Study	n	Valve type	Approach	Ischemic defects	Median number of lesions	Cognitive/neurologic assessment	Cognitive/neurologic assessment results	Stroke
Kahlert et al.[6]	32	Edwards SAPIEN (n = 22)	TF	Edwards: 86%	Edwards: 4 (2.1–6.0)	NIHSS, MMSE, mRS	No change	Overall: 0%
		CoreValve (n = 10)		CoreValve: 80%	CoreValve: 2.6 (0.3–4.9)			
Ghanem et al.[7]	22	CoreValve	TF	73%	2.5 (1.0–5.5)	NIHSS, NSE	Neurologic impairment: 3 (10%)	3.6%
					Overall: 3 (2–8)			Overall: 3.3%
Rodes-Cabau et al.[9]	60	Edwards SAPIEN	TF (n = 29) TA (n = 31)	TF: 66% TA: 71%	TF: 3 (1–7) TA: 4 (2–9)	NIHSS, MMSE	No change	TF: 3.4% TA: 3.2%
Fairbairn et al.[10]	31	CoreValve	TF	77%	2 (1–5)	NIHSS	No change	6.0%
Arnold et al.[8]	25	Edwards SAPIEN	TA	68%	N/A	Standardized clinical assessment	Neurologic impairment: 5 (20%)	4.0%

TA, transapical; TF, transfemoral; NIHSS, National Institutes of Health Stroke Scale; MMSE, Mini-Mental State Examination; mRS, modified Rankin Scale; NSE, neuron-specific enolase.

however demonstrated new hyperintense lesions in 86% of the Edwards Sapien and 80% of CoreValve TAVI patients. There were significantly fewer patients with new lesions in the control SAVR group (48%, $P = 0.016$). These new lesions were typically identified in both hemispheres reflecting a probable embolic cause. The lesion size was significantly smaller in the TAVI groups compared with the SAVR patients. Three-month follow-up did not reveal any new DW MRI findings or changes in clinical or neurocognitive testing. Indeed, the authors state that 80% of new lesions had no residual signal change, on repeat DW MRI at the three-month interval. Ghanem et al.[7] performed a pilot study involving 22 patients to prospectively assess clinically silent and overt cerebral embolic events in the setting of TF TAVI. Cerebral DW MRI was carried out before, within three days and at three months after valve implantation. Three patients (10%) had a new neurological abnormality on examination post-TAVI, but symptoms resolved in two. At the time of the first post-TAVI neuroimaging study, 73% of patients had new ischemic lesions compared to baseline.

It had been suggested that the transapical (TA) approach may potentially have lower cardioembolic event rates as this method potentially minimizes extensive catheter manipulation within the aortic arch. Arnold et al.[8] performed a similar assessment using cerebral DW MRI in 25 patients undergoing TA TAVI with the Edwards Sapien system. Valve implantation was successful in all, though neurological

abnormalities were evident postprocedure on clinical examination in five patients, one of whom developed a major stroke. Analysis of DW MRI revealed new embolic lesions in 68% of the patients, with more than one lesion in the majority. In those patients with new lesions, the posterior circulation territory was involved in more than 50% of cases. Rodès-Cabau et al.[9] compared the incidence of acute cerebral ischemic injury in those undergoing TAVI (employing the Edwards SAPIEN or SAPIEN XT valve) via the TF and the TA approach. In this multicenter study, 60 patients (TF: 29, TA: 31) underwent cerebral DW MRI before and within six days following TAVI. Additional neurologic and cognitive evaluation was performed at the same intervals as neuroimaging, using the NIHSS and MMSE tests. One patient in each group had clinical evidence of a stroke within 24 hours of valve insertion. Up to 68% of patients had new ischemic lesions on DW MRI post-TAVI, with a median number of three lesions per patient (range: 1–36). Of those with new lesions, 76% were multiple, and 73% and 66% involved both cerebral hemispheres and circulation (anterior and posterior) territories, respectively. Of note, most lesions (91%) were small (<1 cm). There were no significant differences between groups with regard to the incidence of new ischemic lesions between the TF (66%) and TA (71%) approaches. Finally, no interval changes in NIHSS and MMSE test scores were recorded following TAVI. Fairbairn et al.[10] examined quality of life data in addition to performing

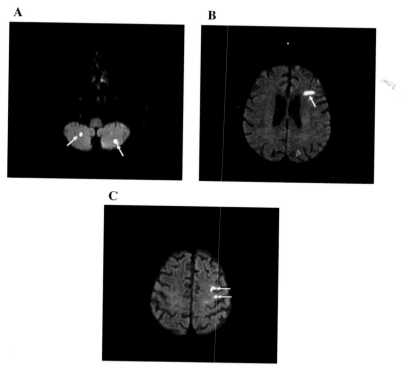

Figure 1. DW MRI images following transapical transcatheter aortic valve implantation (TA-TAVI) in an 83-year-old patient showing multiple acute ischemic lesions in the left and right cerebellum (A, white arrows) and left frontal territory (B and C, white arrows). Reproduced from Rodés-Cabau *et al.*[9] with the permission of the author and publisher.

DW MRI pre- and post-TAVI with the CoreValve system in 31 AS patients. Two (6%) patients were diagnosed clinically with stroke as a consequence of the procedure. DW MRI confirmed up to 26 new ischemic lesions in both of these. Overall new cerebral ischemic lesions were seen in 24 (77%) patients, with the infarcts distributed evenly between both hemispheres. The mean number of new lesions per patient was 4.2 ± 6.5, with a mean infracted tissue volume of 2.05 ± 3.5 mL. The authors demonstrated that increasing age and aortic arch atheroma burden, were independent predictors of new ischemic lesions post-TAVI. General health status and quality of life improved at 30 days post-TAVI, with no functional cognitive decline recorded.

The significance of clinically silent cerebrovascular ischemic events post-TAVI remains unclear. As detailed above DW MRI evaluation has shown that between 68% and 86% of TAVI patients have evidence of acute ischemic insults.[6–10] General population studies have found that the prevalence of silent brain infarcts increases with age and may be as high as 28%, fivefold more common than stroke.[11–13] Al-

though the consequences of silent cerebral ischemia are not fully elucidated, they have been associated with visual defects, motor abnormalities, cognitive decline, and altered mood.[14] Furthermore, they have been shown to indicate an increased risk of subsequent stroke in those with a history of minor stroke and atrial fibrillation (AF).[15] Further studies will have to elucidate the real clinical consequences of these DW MRI defect following TAVI procedures.

TAVI and cerebrovascular events

In the initial experience of TAVI, the rates of procedure-related stroke varied considerably from under 4% to 10%.[16,17] It is likely that outcomes in these small series were influenced by a multitude of factors that go hand in hand with the introduction of a new procedure. These may include an operator-related learning curve with any novel procedure, TAVI system design evolution, in addition to enhanced patient periprocedural clinical management. Following these initial TAVI experiences, several large multicenter registries were carried out, including about 4,000 patients considered

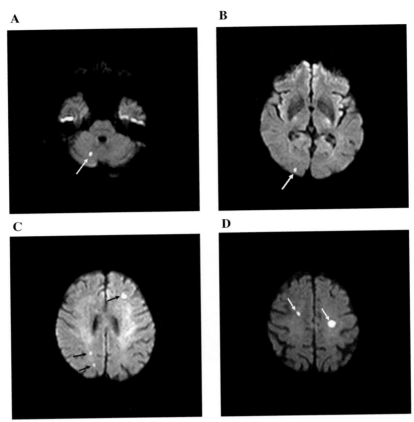

Figure 2. DW MRI images following transfemoral transcatheter aortic valve implantation (TF-TAVI) in an 86-year-old patient showing multiple acute ischemic lesions in the right cerebellum (A, white arrow), right occipital territory (B, white arrow), left frontal and right parietal territories (C, black arrows), and left and right frontal superior territories (D, white arrows). Reproduced from Rodés-Cabau et al.[19] with the permission of author and publisher.

nonoperable, or at very high risk for SAVR. Findings from the eight largest recent multicenter registries and series of TAVI published in the past few years[18–26] are summarized in Table 2. Most patients included in these registries were octogenarians, and had several comorbidities leading to a high-risk profile (mean logistic EuroSCORE >20%). The mean stroke rate reported in these registries was ~3.5%, ranging from 0.6% to 5%. It is important to note that there has been no standardization among these studies, with regard to the definition of cerebrovascular complications associated with TAVI. This may have played a role in the different stroke rates observed among TAVI registries/series. In an effort to standardize data reporting, a recently formed multispeciality committee, the Valve Academic Research Consortium (VARC), drew up guidelines defining recommended clinical endpoints for TAVI studies.[27]

Those in relation to cerebrovascular events are outlined in Table 3. Although most registries and trials have reported major stroke largely in accordance with these VARC guidelines, significant inconsistencies may exist between studies.

The PARTNER trial is, to date, the only prospective randomized trial of TAVI. PARTNER included two differentiated cohorts of patients, those considered to be nonoperable (i.e., comorbidities leading to a predicted risk of 50% or more, of either death by 30 days after surgery, or a serious irreversible morbidity; patients with comorbidities leading to a life expectancy <1 year were excluded; cohort B, n = 358),[28] and those considered to be at high-surgical risk (i.e., predicted risk of operative mortality ≥15% as determined by the trial site surgeon and cardiologist; guideline = STS score ≥10; cohort A, n = 699).[29] The Edwards SAPIEN valve was used in all

Table 2. Overview of large recent TAVI registries/series

Study	Approach	TAVI system	Mean age	Logistic EuroSCORE %	Periprocedure/ 30-days stroke %	30-day mortality	1-year stroke %	1-year survival
Piazza et al.[18] Europe (51 sites) n = 646	TF: 646	CoreValve	TF: 81.0	TF: 23.1 ± 13.8	TF: 1.9	TF: 8.0	N/A	N/A
Rodés-Cabau et al.[19] Canada (6 sites) n = 339	TF: 162 TA: 177	Cribier-Edwards: 57 Edwards SAPIEN: 275 Edwards SAPIEN XT: 7	TF: 83 TA: 80	Overall: 27.7 ± 16.3 TF: 25.8 ± 14.9 TA: 29.4 ± 17.2	Overall: 2.3 TF: 3.0 TA: 1.7	Overall: 10.4 TF: 9.5 TA: 11.3	N/A	Overall: 76 TF: 75 TA: 78
Thomas et al.[20,21] Europe (32 sites) n = 1038	TF: 463 TA: 575	Edwards SAPIEN	TF: 81.7 TA: 80.7	TF: 25.7 ± 14.5 TA: 29.1 ± 16.3	Overall: 2.5 TF: 2.4 TA: 2.6	Overall: 8.5 TF: 6.3 TA: 10.3	Overall: 5.5	Overall: 76.1 TF: 81.1 TA: 72.1
Eltchaninoff et al.[22] France (16 sites) n = 244	TF Edwards: 95 TA Edwards: 71 TF CoreValve: 66 SC CoreValve: 12	Edwards SAPIEN: 166 CoreValve: 78	Overall: 82.3 TF Edwards: 83.2 TA Edwards: 82.1 TF CoreValve: 82.5 SC CoreValve: 75.5	Overall: 25.6 ± 11.4 TF Edwards: 25.6 ± 11.3 TA Edwards: 26.8 ± 11.6 TF CoreValve: 24.7 ± 11.2 SC CoreValve: 24.6 ± 14.5	Overall: 3.6 TF Edwards: 4.2 TA Edwards: 2.8 TF CoreValve: 4.5 SC CoreValve: 0	Overall: 12.7 TF Edwards: 8.4 TA Edwards: 16.9 TF CoreValve: 15.1 SC CoreValve: 8.3	N/A	N/A
Zahn et al.[23] Germany (22 sites) n = 697	TF: 644 SC: 22 TA: 26 Tao: 5	Edwards SAPIEN: 109 CoreValve: 588	Overall: 81.4	Overall: 20.5 ± 13.2	Overall: 2.8	Overall: 12.4	N/A	N/A
Bosmans et al.[24] Belgium (15 sites) n = 328	TF/TA Edwards: 187 TF CoreValve: 141	Edwards SAPIEN: 187 CoreValve: 141	Overall: 83 TF/TA Edwards: 83 TF CoreValve: 82	Overall: 28 ± 16 TF/TA Edwards: 30 ± 16 TF CoreValve: 25 ± 15	Overall: 5.0 TF/TA Edwards: 5.0 TF CoreValve: 4.0	Overall: 11.0 TF/TA Edwards: 12.0 TF CoreValve: 11.0	N/A	TF Edwards: 82 TF/TA Edwards: 63 TF CoreValve: 79
Tamburino et al.[25] Italy (14 sites) n = 663	TF: 599 SC: 64	CoreValve	Overall: 81	Overall: 23.0 ± 13.7	Overall: 1.2	Overall: 5.4	Overall: 2.5	Overall: 85
Moat et al.[26] United Kingdom (25 sites) n = 870	TF: 599 Other approaches: 271	Edwards SAPIEN: 410 CoreValve: 452	Overall: 81.9 TF: 81.7 Other routes: 82.3 CoreValve: 81.3 Edwards: 82.6	Overall: 18.5 (11.7–27.9) TF: 17.1 (11, 25.5) Other routes: 21.4 (14.4, 33.6) CoreValve: 18.1 (11.1, 27.9) Edwards: 18.5 (12.4, 27.7)	Overall: 4.1 TF: 4.0 Other routes: 4.1 CoreValve: 4.0 Edwards: 4.2	Overall: 7.1 TF: 5.5 Other routes: 10.7 CoreValve: 5.8 Edwards: 8.5	N/A	Overall: 78.6 TF: 81.5 Other routes: 72.3 CoreValve: 78.3 Edwards: 79.4

TA, transapical; TF, transfemoral; SC, subclavian; TAO, transaortic.

cases. The primary endpoint was all cause mortality at one year follow-up, and the trial was powered to demonstrate the superiority of TAVI versus medical treatment (including balloon valvuloplasty [BAV]) and the noninferiority of TAVI versus SAVR for the high-surgical risk cohort. The PARTNER trial showed, in the nonoperable cohort, the superiority of TAVI versus medical treatment/BAV (mortality at one-year follow-up of 30.7% vs. 50%, $P < 0.001$), and the noninferiority of TAVI versus SAVR in the

Table 3. VARC stroke definitions

Stroke diagnostic criteria

- Rapid onset of a focal or global neurological deficit with at least one of the following: change in level of consciousness, hemiplegia, hemiparesis, numbness or sensory loss affecting one side of the body, dysphasia or aphasia, hemianopia, amaurosis fugax, or other neurological signs or symptoms consistent with stroke
- Duration of a focal or global neurological deficit ≥24 h; OR <24 h, if therapeutic intervention(s) were performed (e.g., thrombolytic therapy or intracranial angioplasty); OR available neuroimaging documents a new hemorrhage or infarct; OR the neurological deficit results in death
- No other readily identifiable nonstroke cause for the clinical presentation (e.g., brain tumor, trauma, infection, hypoglycemia, peripheral lesion, pharmacological influences)
- Confirmation of the diagnosis by at least one of the following:
  Neurology or neurosurgical specialist

Stroke definitions

- Transient ischemic attack:
New focal neurological deficit with rapid symptom resolution (usually 1–2 h), always within 24 h;
  Neuroimaging without tissue injury
- Stroke:
(diagnosis as above, preferably with positive neuroimaging study)
Minor—modified Rankin score 2 at 30 and 90 days
Major—modified Rankin score 2 at 30 and 90 days

From Ref. 27.

high-risk cohort (mortality at one-year follow-up of 24.2% vs. 26.8%, $P = 0.44$). However, the trial showed a higher rate of cerebrovascular events in the TAVI group with respect to the medical treatment and SAVR groups. A summary of the results regarding the cerebrovascular events in the PARTNER trial at 30-day and at one-year follow-up is shown in Figure 3.

Pathophysiology of cerebroembolic events during TAVI

Consideration of the individual facets of the TAVI procedure highlights the multiple stages during which inadvertent embolic showering of the cerebral circulation may occur, potentially leading to periprocedural acute stroke. Left heart catheterization alone via the TF approach, wherein the stenosed AV is crossed in its retrograde fashion, has been shown to result in cerebroemboli.[30] For instance, Omran et al.[30] described the occurrence of clinically apparent stroke in 3%, and cerebral DW MRI changes consistent with acute ischemic lesions in 22%, following retrograde AV crossing. TA TAVI conceptually may reduce cerebral embolic debris release during transvalvular wire delivery as less manipulation of catheters and wires

is usually needed with this antegrade approach. Several studies employing cerebral DW MRI have shown asymptomatic ischemic lesions due to cardiac catheterization with an incidence ranging from 5% to 22% of the aforementioned work.[30–32] Clinically, overt stroke has been reported after 0.44% of patients undergoing PCI, and occurred in association with diabetes mellitus, hypertension, prior stroke, or renal failure.[33] However, age has been shown to influence this rate, with one study showing a more than doubling of the stroke rate in patients older than 80 years (0.58% vs. 0.23%, $P <$ 0.001).[34] Perhaps of even more relevance to TAVI are the associations between aortic atheroma, aortic scraping during catheter manipulation, and release of microemboli.[35–37] Cerebroemboli may also be gaseous or originate from thrombi formed on the catheter or introducer sheath surface, in addition to displaced endovascular atheroma. The very large sheaths necessary for TAVI make smooth transitioning through the peripheral vasculature especially challenging. Furthermore, even with meticulous catheter preparation and flushing, air emboli are commonly observed using transoesophageal echocardiography.[9] A significant potential also exists with these catheters for air entrainment leading to large gaseous emboli.[38] BAV is an important step during TAVI to facilitate delivery of the undeployed valve. An early study using computed tomography alone described radiographic evidence of new cerebral ischemia in three of 26 patients following BAV.[39] A more recent series looked at outcomes following BAV in 262 high-risk patients (mean logistic EuroSCORE 45.6 ± 21.6), and reported a stroke rate which was close to 2%.[40] TAVI also necessitates at least one-to-two AV dilations depending on the use of self-expandable or balloon-expandable valves, respectively, and this carries the risk of releasing calcific valve particles intra-arterially, which may result in the occurrence of a cerebrovascular event. Kahlert et al.[41] detailed intraoperative transcranial Doppler (TCD) ultrasound findings of both middle cerebral arteries in 46 patients during TAVI (TF: 32, TA: 14). The results of this study showed that though high-intensity transient signals (HITS) can occur almost at any time during the TAVI procedure, the greatest number seem to occur during actual valve positioning and implantation. Similarly Drews et al.[42] performed TCD ultrasonography of both middle cerebral arteries in 50 patients undergoing TA-TAVI. The greatest number of HITS and microembolic signals were detected during BAV and with passage of the undeployed valve. Szeto et al.[43] employed TCD ultrasonography to evaluate 28 patients who underwent TAVI with a balloon-expandable valve by TF or TA approach. The main results of this study showed that most HITS occurred during wire manipulation in the aortic arch and with valve deployment. No significant difference in the number of HITS was seen between TF and TA approaches. These transcranial Doppler studies provide important insight into the mechanisms of cerebral emboli during TAVI procedures, and strongly suggest that most embolic episodes occur during the interaction between the transcatheter valve prosthesis and the native aortic valve (valve positioning and deployment). This might explain the lack of observed differences in adverse cerebrovascular events, between the TF and TA approaches. This is despite the operator, when using the TA approach, being able to minimize the manipulation of large catheters in the ascending aorta, and to avoid their transition through the aortic arch. Miller et al.[44] recently reported the results of a PARTNER substudy primarily focusing on neurological events. In-

terestingly, the acute cerebrovascular events were associated with smaller valve areas, which are usually associated with a higher degree of valve calcification.[45,46]

Another potentially important contributor to ischemic brain injury during TAVI is hypoperfusion, which may occur at a number of stages during valve implantation. For instance, BAV and deployment of the balloon-expandable valves are routinely done during rapid right ventricular pacing to prevent device ejection. These episodes may induce cerebral ischemia in watershed territories, as well as impairing the washout of dislodged microemboli. Indeed, it has been shown that the combination of hypoperfusion and cerebral emboli often coexist in a number of clinical situations such as cardiac surgery.[47] Transitory poor cerebral perfusion may accentuate the microembolic ischemic effects by reducing the effectiveness of the circulation to washout debris promptly.

From the data that currently exists, it appears that a significant risk of stroke persists beyond the immediate periprocedural period. Rodés-Cabau et al.[19] found that periprocedural stroke was diagnosed in two patients (0.6%), whereas a further six (1.7%) patients suffered a stroke between this time point and 30 days. Analysis of the PARTNER trial demonstrated that 27% (n = 3) of strokes occurred within 24 hours, 55% (n = 6) between days 1–5 and 18% (n = 2) one week post-TAVI.[28] Combined data from the Canadian Registry[19] and PARTNER Cohort B[28] (nonoperable patients with severe AS), reveals that 13 of the 22 stroke events that were reported by 30 days in both of these studies, occurred in the 24-hour to 30-day period post-TAVI (Fig. 3). The variability in the timing of stroke occurrence following TAVI suggests that mechanisms other than catheter-induced cerebral embolization or native valve dilation resulting in embolic debris may be at play. Miller et al.[44] showed that cerebrovascular events occurring after the periprocedural period, were mostly related to higher atherosclerotic burden, with patients who suffered late strokes exhibiting higher rates of extensive peripheral arterial disease which had necessitated a TA approach. In addition, these patients were found to have had a higher rate of stroke in the 6–12 month period before their TAVI procedure.

A further potential etiological factor of stroke is TAVI-associated AF. Recently, our group described

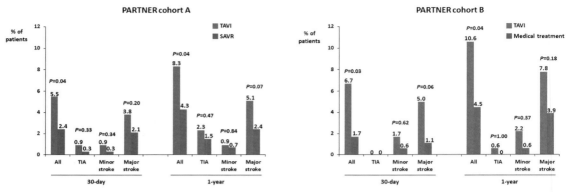

Figure 3. Cerebrovascular events in the PARTNER trial at 30 days and at one-year follow-up in (A) the high-risk cohort (cohort A),[29] and (B) the nonoperable cohort (cohort B).[28]

the incidence and prognostic value of new-onset AF after TAVI.[48] In a series of 138 patients undergoing TAVI, almost 32% developed new-onset AF at a median of 48 h postvalve implantation. A higher incidence was seen in the TA approach (37% vs. 15.8%, $P = 0.019$), and new-onset AF was associated with a higher stroke/systemic embolism rate at 30 days (13.6% vs. 3.2%, $P = 0.021$). Importantly, new-onset AF was found to be the strongest predictor of cardioembolic events occurring after the first 24 h following the procedure, suggesting again, that the mechanisms of acute (<24 h) versus subacute (>24 h) stroke post-TAVI are probably different. Finally, given the baseline profile of TAVI patients, it would appear that their elevated risk of stroke intraoperatively and beyond the periprocedural period may be influenced by several non-TAVI related characteristics. For instance, intraoperative and postoperative stroke rates were found to be both increased by older age, small body surface area, previous stroke, preoperative AF, and use of hypothermic circulatory arrest, in a large series of isolated or repeat CABG.[49] In their analysis of 45,432 patients at a single institution, Tarakji *et al.* found an intraoperative stroke risk of 0.87% (95% CI, 0.71–1.1%) and a postoperative risk of 1.5% (95% CI, 1.3–1.7% [168/11,297]) for those 70 years and older. Similarly, data from SAVR has shown that risk factors such as age >75 years at time of surgery, diabetes mellitus, previous stroke, and carotid artery stenosis increase adverse cerebrovascular event rates during long-term follow-up.[50] Patients without these risk factors had cerebrovascular event rates of 1.37% per

patient-year versus 5.18% per patient-year in those with more than one risk factor.

Prognostic value of cerebrovascular events following TAVI

Data from non-TAVI patients show that severe stroke carries a grave prognosis, with a 30-day mortality rate of approximately 58% in those requiring mechanical ventilation.[51] Also, several studies have demonstrated the poor outcomes of patients who suffer a stroke following a cardiovascular intervention. Melby *et al.*[52] examined outcomes in 245 octogenarians who underwent SAVR alone or with CABG. Patients who suffered a perioperative stroke had significantly higher 30-day mortality rates (38% vs. 9%; OR, 11.3; 95% CI, 1.7 to 75.1; $P = 0.019$). Tarakji *et al.*[49] also showed that post-CABG patients who experienced a stroke, had a significantly higher hospital mortality rate (19% [95% CI, 16–22%) vs. 3.7% [95% CI, 3.1–4.5%], $P < 0.001$), which persisted after propensity adjustment for preoperative factors. Furthermore, they were more likely to require prolonged ventilatory assist (44% 95% CI, 32–57% [31/70]) vs. 15% (95% CI, 12–20% [53/343], $P = 0.001$), and management in an intensive care setting (median, 120 vs. 48 h; $P < 0.001$). Higher rates of renal failure (13%; 95% CI, 11–16% [92/705]) vs. 4.3% (95% CI, 3.6%–5.1% [122/2820], $P < 0.001$) and greater postoperative (median, 14 vs. 7 days; $P < 0.001$) lengths of stay were also seen in stroke patients.

Stroke arising from catheter-based interventions is also a potentially catastrophic event. Hamon

Table 4. Embolic protection devices

Device	Approach	Device positioning	Mechanism of action	Pore size	Catheter size
Embrella	Radial	Aortic arch (covering brachiocephalic and left carotid, arteries)	Deflection of embolic material	100 μm	6F
SMT	Femoral	Aortic arch (covering brachiocephalic, left carotid, and left subclavian arteries)	Deflection of embolic material	~200 μm	9F
Claret Medical	Radial	Brachiocephalic trunk Left common carotid (covering brachiocephalic and left carotid arteries)	Capture of embolic material	140 μm	6F

et al.[37] demonstrated an increased relative risk of mortality of 9.95 (95% CI 5.73–17.27, $P < 0.00001$) in pooled data analysis evaluating PCI-related stroke. Although the corresponding data for TAVI-associated stroke remains very limited, Tamburino et al. found that intraprocedural stroke was a predictor of increased mortality (HR 15.76, CI 3.27–75.9, $P = 0.001$), in a study of 663 patients undergoing CoreValve TAVI.[25]

Prevention of TAVI-associated cerebrovascular ischemic injury

Minimizing the risk of TAVI-related stroke is of paramount importance to the overall success of the procedure. Although there is a paucity of hard data to guide the clinician in this rapidly evolving field, it would appear prudent to attempt to apply knowledge obtained from established percuta-neous and open surgical procedures. Techniques to reduce TAVI-associated stroke begin with the patient's preprocedural assessment. Although potential TAVI patients have by their nature significant risk factors for adverse cerebrovascular events, a thorough evaluation with multimodality imaging may aid risk stratification and guide the approach to valve delivery. For instance, significant atheroma burden in the aortic arch may favor a TA approach, conceptually reducing stroke risk, though this has not been backed up by DW MRI and clinical results to date (as outlined in Tables 1 and 2). Patients are usually pretreated with single (aspirin) or dual (aspirin + clopidogrel) antiplatelet therapy, and strict monitoring of intra-procedural anticoagulation is vital, ensuring the target-activated clotting time is maintained. Cardiac anesthesia plays a vital role in preserving hemodynamic stability and minimizing

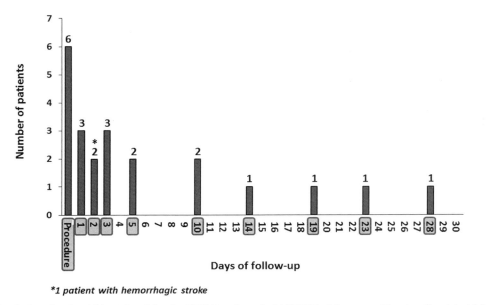

*1 patient with hemorrhagic stroke

Figure 4. Timing of stroke within 30 days following TAVI. Data from the PARTNER trial nonoperable cohort[28] and the Multicenter Canadian Experience.[19]

periods of hypo or hypertension. Over-vigorous BAV before valve insertion should probably be avoided. Similarly, postballoon dilation following valve implantation should also probably be limited to those cases with moderate-to-severe residual paravalvular aortic regurgitation. Meticulous attention must be paid to thorough sheath and catheter flushing, in addition to valve preparation, to reduce thrombus formation and gaseous embolization. Where possible, every effort must be made to employ a technique of smooth transitioning when exchanging and upsizing equipment within the vasculature.

This need to reduce TAVI-associated stroke has spurred significant research and the development of new devices (Table 4). Recently, a potential role for embolic protective devices (EPD) during TAVI has been studied. Though no randomized trials powered for clinical events support the use of mechanical EPD in carotid artery stenting, their use in carotid intervention has become routine.[53] A systematic review included 896 carotid stenting cases with EPD and 2,537 CAS without EPD, and found that EPD usage was associated with lower stroke rates (1.8% vs. 5.5%, $P < 0.001$).[54] Nietlispach et al.[55] described their initial experience with the Embrella Embolic deflector (Edwards Lifesciences, Irvine, California) in three TF TAVI patients (Edwards Sapien valve)

and one BAV patient. This device consists of a nitinol-mounted deflecting membrane composed of heparin-coated polyurethane with a pore size of 100 μm. Initial animal work showed it was effective in deflecting emboli ranging in size from 150 μ to 600 μm away from the carotid circulation.[56] Retrieved particulate matter was reduced in the carotid filtration circuit from 19% (during unprotected aortic injection of prepared human atheroma) to 1.3% with Embrella usage ($P < 0.001$). During the initial clinical study, the device was successfully deployed in all patients via the right radial artery, with the concept of shielding the brachiocephalic and left common carotid arteries from emboli. No clinically overt strokes were found, but postprocedure DW MRI revealed a new ischemic lesion in the BAV patient. Inherent limitations of the device include lack of coverage of the left vertebral arterial system. In addition, the conformity of the device may be affected by different aortic arch types which may impair its ability to defect emboli. Recapture of the device may inadvertently lead to cerebral showering at the end of the procedure. Nonetheless, further refinements to this technique may offer a modality of significantly reducing brain injury.

Another cerebral EPD in evolution is the SMT Embolic Deflection Device (SMT Research and Development Ltd., Herzliya, Israel), which has been designed to deflect debris from all three great aortic arch vessels, and is deployed via the transfemoral route. Like the Embrella system, the Claret dual filter system (Claret Medical Inc, Santa Rosa, California) is deployed via the radial approach but functions by capturing and retaining debris within the proximal brachiocephalic and left common carotid arteries.

It is also worth noting that the risk of stroke, though highest in the periprocedural period, persists following successful TAVI (Fig. 4). The optimal drug therapy post-TAVI also remains unclear, with little data to guide the physician. Most operators routinely continue dual antiplatelet therapy (aspirin and clopidogrel) for a number of months. It is possible that there may be a role for systemic anticoagulation in a role similar to SAVR with bioprosthethic valve. It is conceivable that the displaced valve itself could act as a focus of thrombus formation and lead to subsequent embolization. Current guidelines advise anticoagulation for three months postbioprosthetic SAVR with a target INR of 2.0–3.0 due to the perceived higher risk of thromboembolism during this period.[57,58] However, a number of prospective and retrospective studies concluded that there was no benefit to anticoagulation following bioprosthetic SAVR.[59–61] Furthermore, a large number of TAVI patients, given their comorbidities, are likely to be at an increased risk of hemorrhagic complications and their attendant adverse affects on morbidity and mortality with warfarin therapy. Future studies are necessary to address these issues.

Conclusion

TAVI represents an exciting novel therapy. Continued refinement of the valve systems, procedural techniques, and periprocedural care will aid its successful utilization in patients with severe AS. It is hoped that future studies will address current limitations particularly with regard to reducing procedure related adverse cerebrovascular events. Long-term follow-up data will yield more information about the rate, timing, and outcomes of adverse cerebrovascular event rates in patients undergoing TAVI.

Acknowledgments

We want to thank Mélanie Côté, MSc, from the Quebec Heart and Lung Institute for her help with the preparation of the tables and figures.

Conflict of interest

Dr. Josep Rodés-Cabau is a consultant for Edwards Lifesciences and St-Jude Medical. Dr. Brian Heynes declares no conflict of interest.

References

1. Nkomo, V.T. *et al.* 2006. Burden of valvular heart diseases: a population-based study. *Lancet.* **368:** 1005–1011.
2. Stewart, B.F. *et al.* 1997. Clinical factors associated with calcific aortic valve disease. Cardiovascular Health Study. *J. Am. Coll. Cardiol.* **29:** 630–634.
3. Cribier, A. *et al.* 2002. Percutaneous transcatheter implantation of an aortic valve prosthesis for calcific aortic stenosis: first human case description. *Circulation.* **106:** 3006–3008.
4. Rodés-Cabau, J. 2012. Transcatheter aortic valve implantation: current and future approaches. *Nat. Rev. Cardiol.* **9:** 15–29.
5. Schaff, H.V. 2011. Transcatheter aortic-valve implantation–at what price? *N. Engl. J. Med.* **364:** 2256–2258.
6. Kahlert, P. *et al.* 2010. Silent and apparent cerebral ischemia after percutaneous transfemoral aortic valve implantation: a diffusion-weighted magnetic resonance imaging study. *Circulation.* **121:** 870–878.
7. Ghanem, A. *et al.* 2010. Risk and fate of cerebral embolism after transfemoral aortic valve implantation: a prospective pilot study with diffusion-weighted magnetic resonance imaging. *J. Am. Coll. Cardiol.* **55:** 1427–1432.
8. Arnold, M. *et al.* 2010. Embolic cerebral insults after transapical aortic valve implantation detected by magnetic resonance imaging. *JACC Cardiovasc. Interv.* **3:** 1126–1132.
9. Rodes-Cabau, J. *et al.* 2011. Cerebral embolism following transcatheter aortic valve implantation: comparison of transfemoral and transapical approaches. *J. Am. Coll. Cardiol.* **57:** 18–28.
10. Fairbairn, T.A. *et al.* 2012. Diffusion-weighted MRI determined cerebral embolic infarction following transcatheter aortic valve implantation: assessment of predictive risk factors and the relationship to subsequent health status. *Heart* **98:** 18–23.
11. Price, T.R. *et al.* 1997. Silent brain infarction on magnetic resonance imaging and neurological abnormalities in community-dwelling older adults. The Cardiovascular Health Study. CHS Collaborative Research Group. *Stroke.* **28:** 1158–1164.
12. Di Carlo, A. *et al.* 2000. Frequency of stroke in Europe: a collaborative study of population-based cohorts. ILSA Working Group and the Neurologic Diseases in the Elderly Research Group. Italian Longitudinal Study on Aging. *Neurology.* **54:** S28–S33.
13. Longstreth, W.T., Jr. *et al.* 2001. Frequency and predictors of stroke death in 5,888 participants in the Cardiovascular Health Study. *Neurology.* **56:** 368–375.
14. Vermeer, S.E., W.T. Longstreth, Jr. & P.J. Koudstaal. 2007. Silent brain infarcts: a systematic review. *Lancet Neurol.* **6:** 611–619.
15. EAFT Study Group. 1996. Silent brain infarction in nonrheumatic atrial fibrillation. *Neurology.* **46:** 159–165.

16. Cribier, A. *et al.* 2006. Treatment of calcific aortic stenosis with the percutaneous heart valve: mid-term follow-up from the initial feasibility studies: the French experience. *J. Am. Coll. Cardiol.* **47:** 1214–1223.

17. Grube, E. *et al.* 2007. Percutaneous aortic valve replacement for severe aortic stenosis in high-risk patients using the second- and current third-generation self-expanding CoreValve prosthesis: device success and 30-day clinical outcome. *J. Am. Coll. Cardiol.* **50:** 69–76.

18. Piazza, N. *et al.* 2008. Procedural and 30-day outcomes following transcatheter aortic valve implantation using the third generation (18 Fr) corevalve revalving system: results from the multicentre, expanded evaluation registry 1-year following CE mark approval. *EuroIntervention.* **4:** 242–249.

19. Rodes-Cabau, J. *et al.* 2010. Transcatheter aortic valve implantation for the treatment of severe symptomatic aortic stenosis in patients at very high or prohibitive surgical risk: acute and late outcomes of the multicenter Canadian experience. *J Am Coll Cardiol.* **55:** 1080–1090.

20. Thomas, M. *et al.* 2010. Thirty-day results of the SAPIEN aortic Bioprosthesis European Outcome (SOURCE) Registry: a European registry of transcatheter aortic valve implantation using the Edwards SAPIEN valve. *Circulation.* **122:** 62–69.

21. Thomas, M. *et al.* 2011. One-year outcomes of cohort 1 in the Edwards SAPIEN Aortic Bioprosthesis European Outcome (SOURCE) registry: the European registry of transcatheter aortic valve implantation using the Edwards SAPIEN valve. *Circulation.* **124:** 425–433.

22. Eltchaninoff, H. *et al.* 2010. Transcatheter aortic valve implantation: early results of the FRANCE (FRench Aortic National CoreValve and Edwards) registry. *Eur. Heart J.* **32:** 191–197.

23. Zahn, R. *et al.* 2011. Transcatheter aortic valve implantation: first results from a multi-centre real-world registry. *Eur. Heart J.* **32:** 198–204.

24. Bosmans, J.M. *et al.* 2011. Procedural, 30-day and one year outcome following CoreValve or Edwards transcatheter aortic valve implantation: results of the Belgian national registry. *Interact. Cardiovasc. Thorac. Surg.* **12:** 762–767.

25. Tamburino, C. 2011. Incidence and predictors of early and late mortality after transcatheter aortic valve implantation in 663 patients with severe aortic stenosis. *Circulation.* **123:** 299–308.

26. Moat, N.E. *et al.* 2011. Long term outcomes following transcatheter aortic valve implantation in high risk patients with severe aortic stenosis the UK TAVI registry. *J. Am. Coll. Cardiol.* **58:** 2130–2138.

27. Leon, M.B. *et al.* 2011. Standardized endpoint definitions for transcatheter aortic valve implantation clinical trials: a consensus report from the valve academic research consortium. *J. Am. Coll. Cardiol.* **57:** 253–269.

28. Leon, M.B. 2010. Transcatheter aortic-valve implantation for aortic stenosis in patients who cannot undergo surgery. *N. Engl. J. Med.* **363:** 1597–1607.

29. Smith, C.R. *et al.* 2011. Transcatheter versus surgical aortic-valve replacement in high-risk patients. *N. Engl. J. Med.* **364:** 2187–2198.

30. Omran, H. *et al.* 2003. Silent and apparent cerebral embolism after retrograde catheterisation of the aortic valve in valvular stenosis: a prospective, randomised study. *Lancet.* **361:** 1241–1246.

31. Hamon, M. *et al.* 2006. Cerebral microembolism during cardiac catheterization and risk of acute brain injury: a prospective diffusion-weighted magnetic resonance imaging study. *Stroke.* **37:** 2035–2038.

32. Lund, C. *et al.* 2005. Cerebral emboli during left heart catheterization may cause acute brain injury. *Eur. Heart J.* **26:** 1269–1275.

33. Dukkipati, S. *et al.* 2004. Characteristics of cerebrovascular accidents after percutaneous coronary interventions. *J. Am. Coll. Cardiol.* **43:** 1161–1167.

34. Batchelor, W.B. *et al.* 2000. Contemporary outcome trends in the elderly undergoing percutaneous coronary interventions: results in 7,472 octogenarians. National Cardiovascular Network Collaboration. *J. Am. Coll. Cardiol.* **36:** 723–730.

35. Keeley, E.C. & C.L. Grines. 1998. Scraping of aortic debris by coronary guiding catheters: a prospective evaluation of 1,000 cases. *J. Am. Coll. Cardiol.* **32:** 1861–1865.

36. Khoury, Z. *et al.* 1997. Frequency and distribution of atherosclerotic plaques in the thoracic aorta as determined by transesophageal echocardiography in patients with coronary artery disease. *Am. J. Cardiol.* **79:** 23–27.

37. Hamon, M., J.C. Baron & F. Viader. 2008. Periprocedural stroke and cardiac catheterization. *Circulation.* **118:** 678–683.

38. Berry, C., R. Cartier & R. Bonan. 2007. Fatal ischemic stroke related to nonpermissive peripheral artery access for percutaneous aortic valve replacement. *Catheter. Cardiovasc. Interv.* **69:** 56–63.

39. Davidson, C.J. *et al.* 1988. The risk for systemic embolization associated with percutaneous balloon valvuloplasty in adults. A prospective comprehensive evaluation. *Ann. Intern. Med.* **108:** 557–560.

40. Ben-Dor, I. *et al.* 2010. Complications and outcome of balloon aortic valvuloplasty in high-risk or inoperable patients. *JACC Cardiovasc. Interv.* **3:** 1150–1156.

41. Kahlert, P. *et al.* 2010. cerebral embolization during transcatheter aortic valve implantation (TAVI): a transcranial Doppler study. *Circulation.* **122:** A18122.

42. Drews, T. *et al.* 2011. Transcranial Doppler sound detection of cerebral microembolism during transapical aortic valve implantation. *Thorac. Cardiovasc. Surg.* **59:** 237–242.

43. Szeto, W.Y. 2011. Cerebral embolic exposure during transfemoral and transapical transcatheter aortic valve replacement. *J. Card. Surg.* **26:** 348–354.

44. Miller, C. 2011. Transcatheter (TAVR) versus surgical (AVR) aortic valve replacement: incidence, hazard, determinants, and consequences of neurological events in the PARTNER Trial. Paper presented at: AATS 91st Annual Meeting; May 7–11, 2011; Philadelphia, PA.

45. Messika-Zeitoun, D. *et al.* 2004. Evaluation and clinical implications of aortic valve calcification measured by electron-beam computed tomography. *Circulation.* **110:** 356–362.

46. Cueff, C. *et al.* 2011. Measurement of aortic valve calcification using multislice computed tomography: correlation with haemodynamic severity of aortic stenosis and clinical

implication for patients with low ejection fraction. *Heart.* **97:** 721–726.

47. Caplan, L.R. & M. Hennerici. 1998. Impaired clearance of emboli (washout) is an important link between hypoperfusion, embolism, and ischemic stroke. *Arch. Neurol.* **55:** 1475–1482.

48. Amat-Santos I.J. *et al.* 2012. Incidence, predictive factors and prognostic value of new-onset atrial fibrillation following transcatheter aortic valve implantation. *J. Am. Coll. Cardiol* **59:** 178–188.

49. Tarakji, K.G. *et al.* 2011. Temporal onset, risk factors, and outcomes associated with stroke after coronary artery bypass grafting. *JAMA.* **305:** 381–390.

50. Gulbins, H., I. Florath & J. Ennker. 2008. Cerebrovascular events after stentless aortic valve replacement during a 9-year follow-up period. *Ann. Thorac. Surg.* **86:** 769–773.

51. Holloway, R.G. *et al.* 2005. Prognosis and decision making in severe stroke. *JAMA.* **294:** 725–733.

52. Melby, S.J. *et al.* 2007. Aortic valve replacement in octogenarians: risk factors for early and late mortality. *Ann. Thorac. Surg.* **83:** 1651–1656; discussion 1656–1657.

53. Liapis, C.D. *et al.* 2009. ESVS guidelines. Invasive treatment for carotid stenosis: indications, techniques. *Eur. J. Vasc. Endovasc. Surg.* **37:** 1–19.

54. Kastrup, A. *et al.* 2003. Early outcome of carotid angioplasty and stenting with and without cerebral protection devices: a systematic review of the literature. *Stroke.* **34:** 813–819.

55. Nietlispach, F. *et al.* 2010. An embolic deflection device for aortic valve interventions. *JACC Cardiovasc. Interv.* **3:** 1133–1138.

56. Carpenter, J.P. *et al.* 2011. A percutaneous aortic device for cerebral embolic protection during cardiovascular intervention. *J. Vasc. Surg.* **54:** 174–181 e171.

57. Bonow, R.O. *et al.* 2006. ACC/AHA 2006 guidelines for the management of patients with valvular heart disease: a report of the American College of Cardiology/American Heart Association Task Force on Practice Guidelines (writing committee to revise the 1998 Guidelines for the Management of Patients With Valvular Heart Disease): developed in collaboration with the Society of Cardiovascular Anesthesiologists: endorsed by the Society for Cardiovascular Angiography and Interventions and the Society of Thoracic Surgeons. *Circulation.* **114:** e84–e231.

58. Heras, M. *et al.* 1995. High risk of thromboemboli early after bioprosthetic cardiac valve replacement. *J. Am. Coll. Cardiol.* **25:** 1111–1119.

59. Gherli, T. *et al.* 2004. Comparing warfarin with aspirin after biological aortic valve replacement: a prospective study. *Circulation.* **110:** 496–500.

60. Goldsmith, I. *et al.* 1998. Experience with low-dose aspirin as thromboprophylaxis for the Tissuemed porcine aortic bioprosthesis: a survey of five years' experience. *J. Heart Valve Dis.* **7:** 574–579.

61. Sundt, T.M. *et al.* 2005. Is early anticoagulation with warfarin necessary after bioprosthetic aortic valve replacement? *J. Thorac. Cardiovasc. Surg.* **129:** 1024–1031.

Ann. N.Y. Acad. Sci. ISSN 0077-8923

ANNALS OF THE NEW YORK ACADEMY OF SCIENCES

Issue: *Evolving Challenges in Promoting Cardiovascular Health*

Are we ignoring the dilated thoracic aorta?

Jose M. Castellano,[1,2] Jason C. Kovacic,[1,2] Javier Sanz,[1,2] and Valentin Fuster[1,2,3]

[1]Zena and Michael A. Wiener Cardiovascular Institute, [2]Marie-Josée and Henry R. Kravis Cardiovascular Health Center, Mount Sinai School of Medicine, New York, New York. [3]Centro Nacional de Investigaciones Cardiovasculares (CNIC), Madrid, Spain

Address for correspondence: Valentin Fuster, M.D., Ph.D., Zena and Michael A. Wiener Cardiovascular Institute, Mount Sinai Medical Center, One Gustave L. Levy Place, Box 1030, New York, NY 10029-6574. valentin.fuster@mountsinai.org

The pathophysiology of thoracic aortic aneurysm (TAA) formation involves a complex interplay of genetic predisposition, cardiovascular risk factors, and hemodynamic forces. The medical community has resorted to the use of pharmacologic agents based on weak data transplanted from either abdominal aortic aneurysms (AAAs) or Marfan syndrome. However, aneurysms differ significantly based on their anatomic location and etiology. Epidemiologic and experimental data demonstrate that different genetic and nongenetic risk factors as well as diverse physiologic processes are responsible for the development and progression of sporadic TAA, familial TAA, and AAA. Therefore, these disease processes need to be considered as distinct entities and not hastily grouped together. The extrapolation of data from one aneurysmal disease process to another is still ill-founded and potentially harmful. Clinical trials in TAA are required before medical therapies, such as β-blockers, angiotensin-converting enzyme inhibitors, angiotensin receptor blockers, statins, or macrolide antibiotics, can be recommended.

Keywords: dilated thoracic aorta; thoracic aortic aneurysm; cardiovascular risk factors

Introduction

Thoracic aortic aneurysms (TAAs) significantly increase the risk of aortic dissection or rupture and are an important source of morbidity and mortality. The rise in prevalence of TAA, mainly due to aging of the population and the growing prevalence of hypertension, has led to an increasing interest in the cellular and molecular pathophysiology as well as diagnostic and therapeutic management of patients with aortic pathologies.

The true etiology of aortic aneurysms is probably multifactorial, and the condition occurs in individuals with multiple risk factors. Risk factors for development of TAA include smoking, chronic obstructive pulmonary disease, hypertension, atherosclerosis, male gender, older age, high body mass index, bicuspid or unicuspid aortic valves, and family history. Aortic aneurysms are also more common in men than in women. In addition, several genetic syndromes with a predisposition for TAAs have been identified. Some TAAs are due to an inheritance of a predisposition for the disease, termed familial TAA syndrome, and others remain idiopathic.

Much of the data regarding the use of pharmacologic agents in the management of aortic aneurysms have been generated from studies of patients with abdominal aortic aneurysm (AAA) or with Marfan syndrome. Extrapolation of these data to TAA is controversial, as several differences exist between TAA and AAA that encumber the ability to apply data from one disease process to another (Table 1). The epidemiology of each is distinct, with a fourfold greater prevalence of AAA compared with TAA and a similar imbalance in the incidence of aneurysm rupture.[1] Available data have consistently shown that whereas atherosclerotic risk factors, such as male gender, age, smoking, and hypertension, are strongly associated with AAA, genetic predisposition seems to play a larger role in TAA.[2,3]

Moreover, the etiology of TAA influences the site of its occurrence in the aorta. Most surgically resected TAAs involve the ascending aorta. In a series of 513 ascending TAAs at the Mayo Clinic, 13% of patients had inherited connective tissue disease,

doi: 10.1111/j.1749-6632.2012.06493.x

Table 1. Differences among TAA, AAA, and Marfan syndrome

	TAA	AAA	Marfan
Prevalence	1.25%	5%	1 in 10,000
Risk factors	Genetic predisposition, hypertension	Genetic predisposition, age, male gender, hypertension, smoking	Genetic predisposition
Histology	Cystic medial necrosis	Inflammatory infiltrate, VSMC apoptosis	Cystic medial necrosis
Rate of expansion and rupture	+	++	+++

ABBREVIATIONS: TAA, thoracic aortic aneurysm; AAA, abdominal aortic aneurysm; VSMC, vascular smooth muscle cell. Reproduced with permission from Ref. 1.

mostly Marfan syndrome;[4] 25% had bicuspid aortic valve (BAV) with noninflammatory TAA; 11% had aortitis; and the remaining 51% had idiopathic noninflammatory aneurysms, with approximately 60% of this last group of patients being hypertensive. Atherosclerosis accounts for only 1% of ascending TAAs;[4] however, 90% of descending TAAs are atherosclerotic, with the remaining 10% being chronic dissections.[5] Descending TAAs are less frequently resected than are ascending TAAs, as they are often treated medically (especially chronic dissections).

TAAs are classified in accordance with the portion of aorta involved: the ascending thoracic aorta, the arch, or the descending thoracic aorta. This anatomic distinction is important because the etiology, natural history, and treatment of thoracic aneurysms vary for each of these segments. Aneurysms of the descending aorta are most common, followed by aneurysms of the ascending aorta; aneurysms of the arch occur less often. In addition, descending aortic thoracic aneurysms may extend distally to involve the abdominal aorta and create a thoracoabdominal aortic aneurysm. Sometimes, the entire aorta may be ectatic, with localized aneurysms seen at sites in both the thoracic and abdominal aorta. Interestingly, TAAs are less common than aneurysms of the abdominal aorta.

Regarding dissecting aneurysms, the DeBakey and Stanford classifications are the two most widely used methods of describing the types of dissection. In the DeBakey classification, there are three types of dissection: types I, II, and III. Dissections are classified on the basis of the origin and extent of the

dissecting process. Type III dissections are further divided into IIIa and IIIb. Type IIIa refers to dissections that originate distal to the left subclavian artery but extend proximally and distally, mostly above the diaphragm. Type IIIb refers to dissections that originate distal to the left subclavian artery, extend only distally, and may extend below the diaphragm.[6] In the Stanford system, type A signifies involvement of the ascending aorta, with or without involvement of the arch or the descending aorta (regardless of the site of the primary intimal tear). Type B represents all others, or dissections that do not involve the ascending aorta (Fig. 1).[5]

Epidemiology

Given the indolent nature of TAAs, the true incidence of aneurysm disease is hard to estimate. On the other hand, lethal thoracic aortic dissections are also often misdiagnosed as myocardial infarctions.[7] The widespread use of imaging techniques in the current era has led to the earlier recognition of TAAs, permitting the identification of more patients. Determining whether the apparent increase in number of patients seen with TAA is due to increased detection or to a genuine increase in the incidence of this disease has become a challenge. However, recent evidence suggests the latter.[2]

Data available from population-based studies estimate the incidence of TAAs to be around 10.4 cases per 100,000 person-years.[8] According to the Centers for Disease Control and Prevention death certificate data, diseases of the aorta and its branches account for 43,000–47,000 deaths annually in the United States.[9] Aortic aneurysm disease is the 18th most common cause of death in all individuals and the

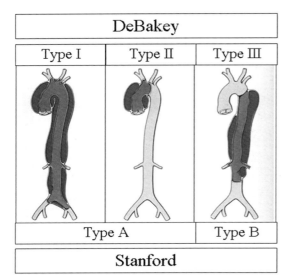

Figure 1. Classification of thoracic aortic dissection.[5]

15th most common in individuals older than age 65 years.[10] Although findings from autopsy series vary widely, the prevalence of TAAs probably exceeds 3–4% in individuals older than 65 years. The incidence of aortic disease is certain to increase both as a result of progressive aging of the population and its associated rise in hypertension prevalence.

Clinical classification of TAAs

The surge in understanding of the molecular mechanisms leading to TAAs as well as the identification of some genes associated with familial TAAs has further improved our knowledge of the disease and aided its classification. TAAs are classified as syndromic, familial, or sporadic.

Nonfamilial syndromic TAAs
Syndromic TAAs are defined as aneurysms that occur in conjunction with a range of associated anomalies affecting various body systems. TAAs are a main feature of some syndromes, namely Marfan syndrome, Loeys-Dietz syndrome, and Ehler-Danlos syndrome (EDS). In other cases, such as BAV syndrome and Turner syndrome, TAAs are a possible manifestation.

Marfan syndrome. Marfan syndrome is a well-defined, autosomal-dominant disorder that involves skeletal, ocular, dural, and cardiovascular findings. The diagnostic criteria have recently been modified and are described in the revised Ghent nosology

(Table 2).[11] This more recent revision places more emphasis on the presence of aortic root aneurysm (defined as an aortic size of ≥ 2 Z-score above the normal range) and ectopic lentis as the predominant clinical features of the disease. The presence of family history of Marfan syndrome only requires one of the following to definitively make the diagnosis: an aortic root aneurysm, ectopic lentis, a pathogenic fibrillin-1 (FBN-1) mutation, or systemic features on physical exam. In the absence of a family history, establishing the diagnosis requires the presence of an aortic aneurysm and one of the following: ectopic lentis, pathogenic FBN-1 mutation, or systemic features. Alternatively, diagnosis can be made by the combination of aortic enlargement not meeting Z-score ≥ 2 with both ectopic lentis and FBN-1 mutation.

Typically, the aortic dilation seen in Marfan syndrome is localized to the aortic root but may extend into the ascending aorta and is associated with an accelerated growth rate (up to 0.2–0.3 cm/year) as compared with degenerative aneurysms. Defects in the FBN-1 gene have been found to lead to excess transforming growth factor beta (TGF-β) signaling and subsequent increased tissue degradation and weakening of the aortic wall.[12,13] Histologically, the aortic tissue in patients with Marfan syndrome has a fraction of the elastin of normal aortas and increased elastin fragmentation. The end result of these processes predisposes patients with Marfan syndrome to a high risk of aortic complications at a relatively young age. The criteria for operative repair in these cases are generally more aggressive than in patients with degenerative aneurysms. In many cases, the aortic valve is morphologically normal and may be able to be resuspended/reimplanted at the time of aortic repair.[14]

Loeys-Dietz syndrome. Loeys-Dietz, a recently described syndrome, involves defects in TGF-β receptors (TGF-βR) 1 or 2. Phenotypic characteristics include hypertelorism, cleft palate, or split uvula, along with some shared characteristics with Marfan syndrome. Patients with this syndrome are at high risk at a young age for aortic dilation, rupture, or dissection. For this reason, very early operative intervention is recommended at ascending aortic diameters of ≥ 4.2 cm by transesophageal echocardiography (TEE) or ≥ 4.4–4.6 cm by computed tomography (CT).[15,16]

Table 2. Revised Ghent criteria for diagnosis of Marfan syndrome[11]

Without family history	With family history
Aortic dissection or Z-score ≥ 2 + ectopia lentis	Aortic dissection or Z-score ≥ 2 in adults, ≥ 3 in children *or*
Aortic dissection or Z-score ≥ 2 + *FBN-1* mutations	ectopia lentis *or*
Aortic dissection or Z-score ≥ 2 + systemic score ≥ 7 points	systemic score ≥ 7 points
Ectopia lentis + *FBN-1* mutations with aortic involvement but Z-score ≤ 2	

Ehlers-Danlos syndrome. EDS is another connective tissue disorder that is characterized by skin hyperelasticity and hypermobile joints, and that can be classified into 11 types. Patients with vascular EDS (type 4) represent a rare but extremely high risk group. Vascular EDS is an inherited connective tissue disease that results from a defect in type III procollagen due to mutations in the COL3A1 gene. Vascular EDS affects 1 in 5–20,000 births. Vascular and connective tissue integrity is markedly impaired, and subsequently, these patients can have significant complications including gastrointestinal complications and uterine rupture in pregnancy. The vascular tissue in these patients is very weak and difficult to safely manipulate in the operating room, even in experienced hands. These patients require specialized care.

BAV syndrome. A significant clinical association with TAA with or without dissection is congenitally BAV. BAV disease is the most common cardiovascular malformation in humans (1–2%). In addition to valvular abnormalities, BAV syndrome can present with various left heart lesions, such as hypoplastic left hearts, arch hypoplasia, and aortic coarctation.[17] TAAs affect about 40% of patients with BAV syndrome and are thought to be associated with increased risk of dissection and rupture.[18] It has been shown that BAV and TAA can occur independently in individuals from families where BAV is manifest.[19] Moreover, a study of 13 families of probands presenting with combined BAV and TAA strongly suggests that BAV-TAA syndrome follows an autosomal-dominant pattern of inheritance.[20]

Familial nonsyndromic TAAs

Although most non-Marfan TAAs are sporadic, familial aggregation studies have suggested a higher prevalence in first-degree relatives. Familial nonsyndromic TAAs follow a familial pattern of inheri-

tance, often autosomal-dominant, with decreased penetrance and variable expression.[21] In a large study of 470 patients with TAAs and no history of Marfan syndrome, family history studies found an inherited pattern in 21.5% of patients.[22] In over 75% of families with multiple affected members, the disease is inherited in an autosomal-dominant manner. Interestingly, an increased risk of abdominal aortic, cerebral, and other aneurysms exists.

The incidence of TAAs in first-degree relatives of patients with isolated TAAs is 11–19%.[23] Although six different genetic loci have been recognized in families with familial nonsyndromic TAAs, only three genes have been identified: TGF-βR2 in TAA2, ACTA2 in TAA4, and MYH11 in familial TAA and patent ductus arteriosus. Studies to identify the specific genes involved in the pathogenesis of these different TAAs are in progress.

Sporadic TAAs

Sporadic TAAs occur in isolation and do not show any familial transmission. The precise cellular and molecular mechanisms remain poorly understood. Sporadic TAAs can also originate in the setting of a broad variety of autoimmune diseases (such as giant cell arteritis, Takayasu arteritis, rheumatoid arthritis, or Reiter syndrome), and infectious disorders (syphilis or tuberculosis) as well as traumatic conditions. Little is known about the precise pathophysiological mechanisms involved in sporadic TAAs. Most of these aneurysms are characterized by inflammatory and immune cell infiltration in the aortic wall, accompanied by matrix degradation and elastin fragmentation.

Pathophysiology

Molecular physiology

A balanced composition of vascular smooth muscle cells and extracellular matrix (ECM) proteins, as found in the medial layer of the aorta, seems critical for preserving its functional properties, particularly its mechanical compliance with pulsatile blood flow. Metabolic imbalance resulting in excessive ECM degradation could be key in progressive aortic wall deterioration that leads to expansion or rupture.[24] TGF-β1 has a central role in cardiac and vascular morphogenesis and in maintaining ECM homeostasis, and is now recognized as a key component in the pathogenesis of TAAs. TGF-β1 has been shown to lead to matrix degradation through increased production of plasminogen activators and release of matrix metalloproteinases (MMPs) 2 and 9.[25] MMPs and their tissue inhibitors (TIMPs), constitute a group of more than 20 zinc-dependent proteolytic enzymes that are instrumental in ECM metabolism and aortic wall remodeling, and are potentially implicated in the development of aneurysms or dissection.[26,27] Murine models without the MMP-9 gene have demonstrated attenuated TAA formation.[28] Moreover, recent human studies have shown high local concentrations of MMP-8 and MMP-9 in ruptured abdominal aortic aneurysm samples with subsequent rapid expansion and rupture.[29] Increased MMP-9 and MMP-2 levels and low tissue inhibitor of metalloproteinase expression have also been observed in patients with thoracic aortic disease.[30]

The characterization of the molecular pathogenesis in Marfan syndrome has helped shed light on the mechanisms that govern TAAs and lead to aortic dissections. The majority of cases of Marfan syndrome are caused by a mutation in the FBN-1 on chromosome 15 (15q21.1).[31] FBN-1 is a matrix glycoprotein widely distributed in elastic and nonelastic tissues. FBN-1 monomers associate to form complex extracellular macroaggregates—termed microfibrils—which form part of elastic fibers. Interestingly, FBN-1 acts as potent regulator of TGF-β1 bioavailability, and reduced or mutated forms of FBN-1 have been shown to stimulate release of sequestered TGF-β1 and an increase in its activity. The various manifestations of Marfan syndrome are today considered to be the result of an overall abnormality in the homeostasis of the ECM, in which altered expression of FBN-1 leads to alterations in the mechanical properties of tissues, increased TGF-β activity and signaling, and loss of cell–matrix interactions.[32] The abnormal homeostasis is thought to result in vascular remod-

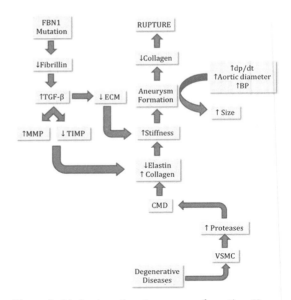

Figure 2. Mechanism of aortic aneurysm formation. Homeostasis of the aortic wall is maintained by several enzymes and growth factors that include TGF-β, matrix metalloproteinases (MMPs) and tissue inhibitors of matrix metalloproteinases (TIMPs). The relative concentration of active MMPs and TIMPs determines net proteolytic activity. The first degenerative change noted in the aging aorta is cystic medial degeneration (CMD), an accumulation of mucopolysaccharide cysts within the aortic media that damages the elastin skeleton and leads to loss of VSMCs and that may disrupt the lamellar structure of the media. An imbalance between MMP and TIMP activity leads to proteolysis and aortic wall weakening. Elastin degradation fragments, in addition to inflammatory cytokines, chemokines, and prostaglandin derivates, promote leukocyte recruitment that perpetuates and amplifies the degradation cycle. Together, the inflammatory milieu, elastic fiber fragmentation, medial attenuation, and decreased collagen reduce the structural integrity of the aorta and ultimately result in aneursymal dilatation (adapted with permission from Ref. 1).

eling, characterized by an exaggerated elastolysis as a result of overexpression of MMP-2 and MMP-9 (Fig. 2).[33]

Mechanical regulation

Circumferential wall tension in the aorta is directly related to the transmural pressure (intravascular pressure minus the extravascular wall pressure) and the radius of the vessel, and inversely proportional to wall thickness (Laplace's law). Thus, increases in aortic diameter or arterial pressure increase wall stress and the risk of aneurysm enlargement, rupture, or dissection. Moreover, not only the absolute level of intraluminal pressure levels but also its rate

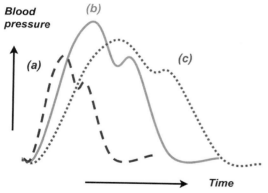

Figure 3. Diagram of aortic pressure. Curve *a*, the administration of a vasodilator agent, such as nitroprusside; curve *b*, the baseline state; curve *c*, β-blockade administration. Note the increase in d*p*/d*t* (slope of the ascending portion of the curve) with vasodilators despite a reduction in mean pressure, an effect that may be deleterious in the setting of aortic dissection (reproduced with permission).

of change over time (d*p*/d*t*; Fig. 3) influence the probability of mechanical complications (see later). Therefore, wall stress alone as a predictor of adverse events is limited in aneurysmal tissue, as some of these physical assumptions may not relate to diseased segments.

Principles of imaging

In the past two decades, survival has improved for patients with acute aortic syndromes or TAAs as a result of technological advances in diagnostic modalities. Current diagnostic techniques for both acute aortic syndromes and TAAs centers around the use of CT, TEE, magnetic resonance imaging (MRI), and, less commonly today, invasive aortography. These four techniques provide variable information as to the site of origin, extent of dissection, classification of dissection, surrounding areas of hemorrhage if applicable, and other pathologic sequelae of the dissection.

Computed tomography

The sensitivity of CT scanning approaches for the detection of both type A and type B TAA. Spiral CT angiography is currently the most frequently used modality worldwide for diagnosing TAA; in nearly two-thirds of patients, it is the first diagnostic tool in making the diagnosis. Similarly, CT angiography is often used to determine the degree of aneurysmal dilatation (Fig. 4). CT scanning has

several limitations. There may be artifacts in the ascending aorta due to cardiac motion, although this can be avoided by the use of electrocardiographic triggering which additionally allow for evaluation of coronary involvement. Streak artifacts may arise from implanted devices and reduce image quality. In addition, the iodinated contrast load ranges from 80 to 120 mL per study, which can result in contrast-induced nephropathy in select patients. Specifically in the setting of type A dissection, CT provides limited evaluation of associated abnormalities in aortic valve function.

MRI

MRI is an acceptable alternative to CT in stable patients with suspected thoracic aortic disease. Excellent anatomic detail and some information on valvular function are available from MRI. A comprehensive MR examination of the thoracic aorta may include many components, including black blood imaging to evaluate aortic morphology and size and aortic wall contour, as well as noncontrast and contrast-enhanced MR angiography using gadolinium-based agents to evaluate the vessel lumen (Fig. 5). The lack of ionizing radiation can make MRI a useful tool for long-term surveillance of TAA, particularly in younger individuals where

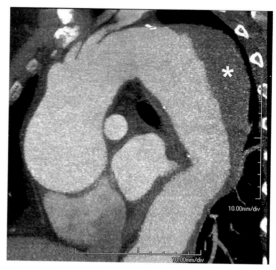

Figure 4. Sagittal maximum intensity projection of a CT angiogram performed in a patient with a diffusely aneurysmal thoracic aorta. There is extensive mural thrombus in the descending segment (asterisk).

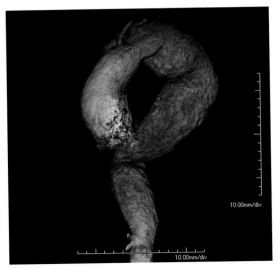

Figure 5. Volume-rendered reconstruction of a contrast-enhanced magnetic resonance angiogram of the aorta, demonstrating a large thoracoabdominal aneurysm.

the accumulated potential cancer risk from repeated imaging is important.

Computational imaging

The recent development of computational fluid dynamics and structural mechanics for the assessment of the aortic root has allowed the creation of patient-specific models that estimate wall shear stress and tensile stress along the aortic root (Fig. 6).[32] These estimations take into account the individual properties of the aorta, which can vary considerably even between patients whose disease shares a similar etiology. In this manner, a tailored evaluation of a patient's risk of aortic complications then becomes possible, which may allow for individualized therapeutic guidance in the future.

Principles of management

With increased understanding of the pathophysiologic processes that are involved in aneurysm formation, greater attention is being given to evaluating pharmacologic interventions that may slow or arrest aneurysm formation. However, although promising results have been seen with the use of renin-angiotensin system blockade, other medical therapies have not proved to be effective.

β-blockers

Medical therapy aimed at reducing wall tension through use of β-adrenergic blockade has its basis from a seminal work by Prokop and colleagues,[34] demonstrating that the pulsatile nature of the cardiac cycle places significant strain on the aorta, especially within its first 2 cm. Pulsatile flow, characterized by a change in pressure over time or dp/dt, contributes to the progression of aortic dissections (see Fig. 3), whereas nonpulsatile flow does not. Because of their favorable effects on dp/dt,[1] β-blockers have become a cornerstone of the medical management of aortic dissection. However, the theoretical benefits of β-blocker therapy for TAA have not been proven clinically. No data support their use in TAA with the possible exception of patients with Marfan syndrome and the recently proven preventive effects of celiprolol (a β1-adrenoceptor blocker with β2-adrenoceptor agonism) in patients with vascular EDS.[35] Together, these data do not support the use of β-blocker therapy in patients with TAA.

Statins

Therapy with 3-hydroxy-3-methylglutaryl-coenzyme A reductase inhibitors (statins) disrupts many of the inflammatory pathways critical in the development of aortic aneurysms. In addition to their lipoprotein-reducing properties, statins have a number of effects called pleiotropic effects. For instance, they reduce oxidative stress by blocking the effects of reactive oxygen species on aneurysms. This effect is independent of their lipid-lowering properties and statins achieve these results through suppressing the NADH/NADPH oxidase system. In a study specifically focusing on tissue samples from patients with TAA, higher levels of reactive oxygen species were seen in aneurysmal tissue than in nonaneurysmal tissue, especially in areas of macrophage and monocyte infiltration.[36] The investigators also observed that expression of p22phox, a component of the oxidase that is responsible for the generation of reactive oxygen species, was reduced in tissue samples from patients who received an angiotensin II receptor blocker or a statin, suggesting that both agents may have a role in inhibiting aneurysm formation.

Aneurysm expansion rate has also been shown to be reduced in AAA patients on statins in observational studies,[37] but the largest study to date failed to

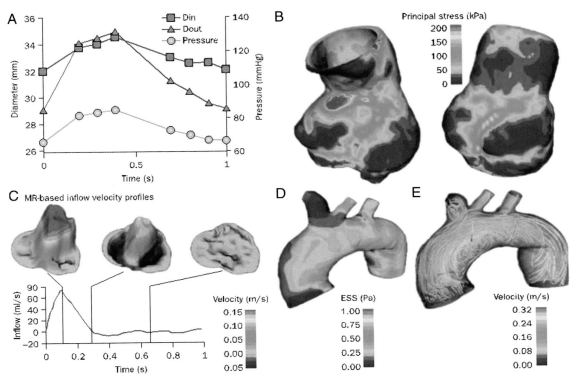

Figure 6. Computational modeling of structural and fluid mechanics in the aortic wall of a patient with aortic root dilatation. Structural mechanical analysis of the aortic root shows (A) the pressure waveform in the aortic root (red) and (B) the tensile stress along the wall of the aortic root. Modeling of fluid mechanics shows (C) flow velocity profiles in the neoaortic root, (D) endothelial shear stress values, and (E) swirling flow velocities in the entire aorta. Reproduced with permission.[32]

show an association between statin prescription and AAA growth rate.[38] At present, however, no clinical data have been able to demonstrate an association between statins and TAA growth.

Antibiotic therapy

Theoretically, the use of antibiotic therapy for aortic aneurysms is justified by evidence of secondary infection with bacteria, such as *Chlamydia pneumoniae* in both atherosclerotic plaques and AAA tissue,[39,40] and by the effectiveness of specific antibiotic agents in attenuating metalloproteinase activity independent of their antibiotic activity.[41] Patients who were randomized to therapy with roxithromycin (300 mg) daily for one month demonstrated slower aneurysm expansion rate than those receiving placebo (1.56 vs. 2.75 mm/year). However, there was no correlation between *C. pneumoniae* titers and inhibition of aneurysm expansion, suggesting that the mechanism of benefit is unrelated

to specific antibiotic activity.[42] Tetracyclines have been shown to antagonize a spectrum of MMPs *in vitro* and in animal models through mechanisms similar to those of endogenous TIMPs, which are independent of their antibiotic activity.[43] Doxycycline prevented the disruption of medial elastin in rodent models and attenuated the dilation of AAA by 33–66% compared with placebo.[44] Although the doses used in these studies (5–30 mg/kg/day) were substantially higher than the usual human dose (1–1.5 mg/kg/day or 200 mg/day), doxycycline (100 mg) administered twice daily in humans achieved similar steady-state plasma concentrations to those required for aneurysm inhibition in rodents. The safety of therapy with doxycycline (200 mg) daily for six months in patients with AAAs has been established in a phase 2 clinical trial, as has its efficacy in reducing MMP expression.[41,45] A randomized trial of 32 patients demonstrated attenuation of aneurysmal growth (from 3.0 to

1.5 mm/year) after three months of treatment with doxycycline (150 mg/day), again with no effect on *C. pneumoniae* titers.[46]

Results of macrolide and tetracycline therapy in animal and preliminary human studies are promising, but the studies have several important limitations in addition to their small size. First, most data were derived from AAA and may not be simply extrapolated to thoracic aorta disease. Second, even if the efficacy of attenuating TAA dilation is established, it must be confirmed that the inhibition of growth does not compromise the structural integrity of aneurysmal tissue such that it is prone to rupture at smaller diameters.

Angiotensin-converting enzyme inhibitors/angiotensin receptor blockers

Angiotensin-converting enzyme inhibitors have been shown to both stimulate and inhibit MMPs and the degradation of ECM in aortic aneurysms. Losartan, an angiotensin I receptor blocker, seems to exert its beneficial effect through blocking TGF-β, thereby reducing matrix degradation in a Marfan syndrome mouse model.[47] The precise mechanisms explaining the role of losartan are still poorly understood. Recently, it has been shown that administration of TGF-β1 neutralizing antibodies to FBN-1 deficient mice reverses the damaging effects associated with TGF-β1 hyperactivity in the aortic wall. Losartan mediates a similar effect. Habashi *et al.* treated seven-week-old FBN-1 deficient mice with documented TAAs with the β-adrenoceptor antagonist propranol or with losartan for a period of six months.[47] Losartan treatment resulted in a significant reduction in aortic size and growth, as well as improved aortic wall architecture.

Indications for surgical repair of TAA

The standard therapy for TAAs is surgical repair. Although the optimal timing of surgery is difficult to predict, most experts advocate surgical intervention when aneurysms of the ascending aorta reach 5.5–6.0 cm in diameter and those of the descending aorta reach 6.0–6.5 cm in diameter. Circumstances in which operative intervention may be required sooner include rapidly expanding aneurysms, associated aortic regurgitation, and/or the presence of aneurysm-associated symptoms. Patients with Marfan syndrome, familial TAA syndrome, or BAV are often referred for surgical repair sooner (i.e., when the aneurysm reaches 4.5–5.0 cm in diameter) be-

Table 3. Indications for surgery in TAAs

Surgical indications in TAAs
≥40 mm with indication for elective aortic valve replacement
≥45 mm in Marfan syndrome
≥50 mm in BAV
≥55 mm for ascending aortic aneurysm
≥60 mm for descending aortic aneurysm
≥70 mm in high-risk comorbidities
Recurrent symptoms, evidence of proximal dissection

cause of their increased risk of aortic dissection and/or rupture at smaller aortic sizes and the relatively low risk of surgery in such patients treated in aortic centers of excellence. The suggested indications for intervention in different TAAs conditions are outlined in Table 3.

Conclusions

The last decade has witnessed the discovery of major findings that have provided valuable insight into the understanding of the cellular and molecular mechanisms leading to TAA formation. Continued research and combined efforts will lead to further elucidation of the inherited and sporadic forms of the disease. This cumulative knowledge will undoubtedly translate into individualized and effective pharmacological treatments oriented toward molecular and genetic mechanisms, allowing for tailored medical and surgical approaches to this serious condition.

Conflicts of interest

The authors declare no conflicts of interest.

References

1. Liao, S.L., S. Elmariah, S. van der Zee, *et al.* 2010. Does medical therapy for thoracic aortic aneurysms really work? Are beta-blockers truly indicated? CON. *Cardiol. Clin.* **28:** 261–269.
2. Elefteriades, J.A. 2008. Thoracic aortic aneurysm: reading the enemy's playbook. *Curr. Prob. Cardiol.* **33:** 203–277.
3. Bickerstaff, L.K. *et al.* 1982. Thoracic aortic aneurysms: a population-based study. *Surgery* **92:** 1103–1108.
4. Homme, J.L. *et al.* 2006. Surgical pathology of the ascending aorta: a clinicopathologic study of 513 cases. *Am. J. Surg. Pathol.* **30:** 1159–1168.

5. Nienaber, C.A. & K.A. Eagle. 2003. Aortic dissection: new frontiers in diagnosis and management: Part I: from etiology to diagnostic strategies. *Circulation* **108:** 628–635.

6. Ramanath, V.S., J.K. Oh, T.M. Sundt 3rd & K.A. Eagle. 2009. Acute aortic syndromes and thoracic aortic aneurysm. *Mayo Clin. Proc.* **84:** 465–481.

7. Acosta, S. *et al.* 2006. Increasing incidence of ruptured abdominal aortic aneurysm: a population-based study. *J. Vasc. Surg.* **44:** 237–243.

8. Clouse, W.D. *et al.* 1998. Improved prognosis of thoracic aortic aneurysms: a population-based study. *JAMA* **280:** 1926–1929.

9. Svensson, L.G. & E.R. Rodriguez. 2005. Aortic organ disease epidemic, and why do balloons pop? *Circulation* **112:** 1082–1084.

10. Elefteriades, J.A. & E.A. Farkas. 2010. Thoracic aortic aneurysm clinically pertinent controversies and uncertainties. *J. Am. Coll. Cardiol.* **55:** 841–857.

11. Loeys, B.L. *et al.* 2010. The revised Ghent nosology for the Marfan syndrome. *J. Med. Genet.* **47:** 476–485.

12. Judge, D.P. & H.C. Dietz. 2008. Therapy of Marfan syndrome. *Annu. Rev. Med.* **59:** 43–59.

13. Canadas, V., I. Vilacosta, I. Bruna & V. Fuster. 2010. Marfan syndrome. Part 1: pathophysiology and diagnosis. *Nature reviews. Cardiology* **7:** 256–265.

14. Canadas, V., I. Vilacosta, I. Bruna & V. Fuster. 2010. Marfan syndrome. Part 2: treatment and management of patients. *Nat. Rev. Cardiol.* **7:** 266–276.

15. Hiratzka, L.F. *et al.* 2010. ACCF/AHA/AATS/ACR/ ASA/ SCA/SCAI/SIR/STS/SVM guidelines for the diagnosis and management of patients with Thoracic Aortic Disease: a report of the American College of Cardiology Foundation/American Heart Association Task Force on Practice Guidelines, American Association for Thoracic Surgery, American College of Radiology, American Stroke Association, Society of Cardiovascular Anesthesiologists, Society for Cardiovascular Angiography and Interventions, Society of Interventional Radiology, Society of Thoracic Surgeons, and Society for Vascular Medicine. *Circulation* **121:** e266–369.

16. Loeys, B.L. *et al.* 2006. Aneurysm syndromes caused by mutations in the TGF-beta receptor. *New Engl. J. Med.* **355:** 788–798.

17. Garg, V. *et al.* 2005. Mutations in NOTCH1 cause aortic valve disease. *Nature* **437:** 270–274.

18. El-Hamamsy, I. & M.H. Yacoub. 2009. A measured approach to managing the aortic root in patients with bicuspid aortic valve disease. *Curr. Cardiol. Rep.* **11:** 94–100.

19. Biner, S. *et al.* 2009. Aortopathy is prevalent in relatives of bicuspid aortic valve patients. *J. Am. Coll. Cardiol.* **53:** 2288–2295.

20. Loscalzo, M.L. *et al.* 2007. Familial thoracic aortic dilation and bicommissural aortic valve: a prospective analysis of natural history and inheritance. *Am. J. Med. Genet. A* **143A:** 1960–1967.

21. Milewicz, D.M. *et al.* 1998. Reduced penetrance and variable expressivity of familial thoracic aortic aneurysms/dissections. *Am. J. Cardiol.* **82:** 474–479.

22. Albornoz, G. *et al.* 2006. Familial thoracic aortic aneurysms and dissections—incidence, modes of inheritance, and phenotypic patterns. *Ann. Thorac. Surg.* **82:** 1400–1405.

23. Pannu, H., V. Tran-Fadulu & D.M. Milewicz. 2005. Genetic basis of thoracic aortic aneurysms and aortic dissections. *Am. J. Med. Genet. C* **139C:** 10–16.

24. Sinha, I. *et al.* 2006. A biologic basis for asymmetric growth in descending thoracic aortic aneurysms: a role for matrix metalloproteinase 9 and 2. *J. Vasc. Surg.* **43:** 342–348.

25. Kim, E.S., M.S. Kim & A. Moon. 2004. TGF-beta-induced upregulation of MMP-2 and MMP-9 depends on p38 MAPK, but not ERK signaling in MCF10A human breast epithelial cells. *Int. J. Oncol.* **25:** 1375–1382.

26. Galis, Z.S. & J.J. Khatri. 2002. Matrix metalloproteinases in vascular remodeling and atherogenesis: the good, the bad, and the ugly. *Circ. Res.* **90:** 251–262.

27. Visse, R. & H. Nagase. 2003. Matrix metalloproteinases and tissue inhibitors of metalloproteinases: structure, function, and biochemistry. *Circ. Res.* **92:** 827–839.

28. Ikonomidis, J.S. *et al.* 2005. Effects of deletion of the matrix metalloproteinase 9 gene on development of murine thoracic aortic aneurysms. *Circulation* **112:** I242–248.

29. Wilson, W.R. *et al.* 2006. Matrix metalloproteinase-8 and -9 are increased at the site of abdominal aortic aneurysm rupture. *Circulation* **113:** 438–445.

30. Ikonomidis, J.S. *et al.* 2006. Expression of matrix metalloproteinases and endogenous inhibitors within ascending aortic aneurysms of patients with Marfan syndrome. *Circulation* **114:** I365–370.

31. Ammash, N.M., T.M. Sundt & H.M. Connolly. 2008. Marfan syndrome: diagnosis and management. *Curr. Probl. Cardiol.* **33:** 7–39.

32. El-Hamamsy, I. & M.H. Yacoub. 2009. Cellular and molecular mechanisms of thoracic aortic aneurysms. *Nat. Rev. Cardiol.* **6:** 771–786.

33. Nataatmadja, M., J. West & M. West. 2006. Overexpression of transforming growth factor-beta is associated with increased hyaluronan content and impairment of repair in Marfan syndrome aortic aneurysm. *Circulation* **114:** I371–377.

34. Prokop, E.K., R.F. Palmer & M.W. Wheat, Jr. 1970. Hydrodynamic forces in dissecting aneurysms. In-vitro studies in a Tygon model and in dog aortas. *Circ. Res.* **27:** 121–127.

35. Ong, K.T. *et al.* 2010. Effect of celiprolol on prevention of cardiovascular events in vascular Ehlers-Danlos syndrome: a prospective randomised, open, blinded-endpoints trial. *Lancet* **376:** 1476–1484.

36. Ejiri, J. *et al.* 2003. Oxidative stress in the pathogenesis of thoracic aortic aneurysm: protective role of statin and angiotensin II type 1 receptor blocker. *Cardiovasc. Res.* **59:** 988–996.

37. Sukhija, R., W.S. Aronow, R. Sandhu, *et al.* 2006. Mortality and size of abdominal aortic aneurysm at long-term follow-up of patients not treated surgically and treated with and without statins. *Am. J. Cardiol.* **97:** 279–280.

38. Ferguson, C.D. *et al.* 2010. Association of statin prescription with small abdominal aortic aneurysm progression. *Am. Heart J.* **159:** 307–313.

39. Nieto, F.J. 2002. Infective agents and cardiovascular disease. *Semin. Vasc. Med.* **2:** 401–415.

40. Lindholt, J.S., H.A. Ashton & R.A. Scott. 2001. Indicators of infection with Chlamydia pneumoniae are associated with expansion of abdominal aortic aneurysms. *J. Vasc. Surg.* **34:** 212–215.

41. Curci, J.A. *et al.* 2000. Preoperative treatment with doxycycline reduces aortic wall expression and activation of matrix metalloproteinases in patients with abdominal aortic aneurysms. *J. Vasc. Surg.* **31:** 325–342.

42. Vammen, S., J.S. Lindholt, L. Ostergaard, *et al.* 2001. Randomized double-blind controlled trial of roxithromycin for prevention of abdominal aortic aneurysm expansion. *Br. J. Surg.* **88:** 1066–1072.

43. Longo, G.M. *et al.* 2005. MMP-12 has a role in abdominal aortic aneurysms in mice. *Surgery* **137:** 457–462.

44. Prall, A.K. *et al.* 2002. Doxycycline in patients with abdominal aortic aneurysms and in mice: comparison of serum levels and effect on aneurysm growth in mice. *J. Vasc. Surg.* **35:** 923–929.

45. Baxter, B.T. *et al.* 2002. Prolonged administration of doxycycline in patients with small asymptomatic abdominal aortic aneurysms: report of a prospective (Phase II) multicenter study. *J. Vasc. Surg.* **36:** 1–12.

46. Mosorin, M. *et al.* 2001. Use of doxycycline to decrease the growth rate of abdominal aortic aneurysms: a randomized, double-blind, placebo-controlled pilot study. *J. Vasc. Surg.* **34:** 606–610.

47. Habashi, J.P. *et al.* 2006. Losartan, an AT1 antagonist, prevents aortic aneurysm in a mouse model of Marfan syndrome. *Science* **312:** 117–121.

Ann. N.Y. Acad. Sci. ISSN 0077-8923

ANNALS OF THE NEW YORK ACADEMY OF SCIENCES

Issue: *Evolving Challenges in Promoting Cardiovascular Health*

Corrigendum for Ann. N.Y. Acad. Sci. 1022: 40–43

Cairns, P. 2004. Detection of promoter hypermethylation of tumor suppressor genes in urine from kidney cancer patients. *Ann. N.Y. Acad. Sci.* **1022:** 40–43.

In the article cited above, the author inadvertently omitted to reference the following article:

Battagli, C., R.G. Uzzo, E. Dulaimi, *et al.* 2003. Promoter hypermethylation of tumor suppressor genes in urine from kidney cancer patients. *Cancer Res.* **63:** 8695–8699.

doi: 10.1111/j.1749-6632.2011.06583.x